PRAISE FOR *SUPERAGING*

"To meet the challenge of population, we do not need a drug—we need a cultural revolution, and this book provides an excellent manifesto for that revolution. We need a new language, a new culture, and a new social reality in which living longer is seen by both individuals and society as an opportunity and a cause for celebration." —Sir Muir Gray, former Chief Knowledge Officer of the National Health Service (UK)

"*SuperAging* moves super fast and never gets old! A riveting ride to a revolutionary new reality of aging, this book sets the pillars to embrace for getting older gracefully and offers a sharp vision of an extended future of sustained good health, well-being, and accomplishment." —Terrence P. O'Brien, MD, Distinguished Professor of Ophthalmology, Bascom Palmer Eye Institute, University of Miami Miller School of Medicine

"We live in a society that treats our seniors as if they are fragile and should be protected behind glass. This book puts the lie to that. I read it. I was a superager; now I'm going to be a SuperAger." —Marshall Cohen, former Deputy Minister of Finance, Government of Canada

"Of the many books on aging, this is one of the most coherent and accessible, sharing insights from lived experience, research, and therapy that will provide the reader with a wealth of information, a healthy game plan, and an optimistic worldview. It approaches successful aging not as a one-size-fits-all enterprise but rather in sync with a precision medicine type of approach that recognizes heterogeneous paths to continued life satisfaction and challenges the reader to discover theirs." —Marsha E. Bates, PhD, Distinguished Professor and Vice Chair of Research, Department of Kinesiology and Health, Rutgers University

"SuperAging is one of the most powerful forces of disruption today. The possibility of 'getting older without getting old' will transform every aspect of our society. This book is your essential guide to what's happening, why it matters, and how to apply it to your own life." —Jim Harris, author of *Blindsided* and *The Learning Paradox*

"Informative, engaging, and encouraging, this book offers more detailed information and resources to the reader than others I've read on aging. As a SuperAger myself, who did not retire until age 75, I found the information here to be both useful and exciting as I look forward to the next 20 years of my life! I've recommended this to my friends and family." —Karen Goldstein, MBA, PhD, former Associate Dean, School of Arts and Sciences, University of Pennsylvania

"This magnificent book is an essential guide for anyone wanting to continue to thrive at any age. It goes well beyond simply living longer and explores how those extra years can become amazingly creative and productive so that aging is not about simply 'surviving' longer but rather thriving longer." —Lisa da Rocha, Executive Coach and expert on Neuro-Transformational leadership

"In a landscape that is cluttered with fads and gimmicks, *SuperAging* is the quintessential guide to rescue you from the perils of poor health and age-related decline." —William Simmons, PhD, Memorial Healthcare System

"*SuperAging* is a compelling guidebook to getting the most out of life as we age. Many readers will have 20 or 30 years ahead after reaching age 65. By drawing on advancements in many fields, the authors persuasively illustrate exciting new opportunities for living those bonus years with vigor. The book deftly addresses seven pillars of aging to help us reimagine and then actualize our prospects for a relevant and optimistic future." —Brent Green, author of *Generation Reinvention*

SUPER AGING

SUPER AGING

GETTING OLDER WITHOUT GETTING OLD

DAVID CRAVIT
AND LARRY WOLF

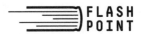

FLASH POINT

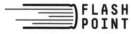

Published by Flashpoint™ Books, Seattle
www.flashpointbooks.com

Produced by Girl Friday Productions

Cover design: David Fassett and Paul Barrett
Project management: Sara Spees Addicott

ISBN (hardcover): 978-1-954854-86-4
ISBN (ebook): 978-1-954854-87-1

Library of Congress Control Number: 2022947538

"You are old, Father William," the young man said,
"And your hair has become very white;
And yet you incessantly stand on your head—
Do you think, at your age, it is right?"
    —Lewis Carroll, *Alice in Wonderland*

Age is just a number and mine is unlisted.
    —Title of a memoir by Manya Nogg, 2015

CONTENTS

INTRODUCTION

In November 2021, Julia "Hurricane" Hawkins set a new world record for the 100-meter dash, clocking in at just under one minute and three seconds.

But isn't that a rather slow time? How can it be a world record?

Julia is 105 years old. In 2017, she set a world record in the 100-to-104-year-old category, only to see that record broken. So she pushed the category to 105-plus, and now she's a world record holder again.

Wait a minute . . . There are *competitions* at this age? There is an actual *category* for 100-to-104-year-olds? And other runners are trying to set records of their own? What's going on here?

Everywhere we look, we see more stories like this—people not only living longer (much longer) but accomplishing things that would have been unthinkable at that same age in previous generations. Just a tiny selection:

- At 99, retired British Army captain Sir Tom Moore raised millions for COVID-beleaguered healthcare workers by walking laps (with the aid of his walker) around his garden. (He died at 100.)

- Prince Philip, who died at 99, didn't announce his retirement from active royal duties until after his 95th birthday. Queen Elizabeth maintained a busy schedule, including receiving incoming prime minister Liz Truss, right up until her passing at age 96.
- In 2022, Republican senator Charles Grassley was reelected to another six-year term at the age of 89.
- Manfred Steiner earned a doctorate in physics from Brown University at the age of 89.
- Betty White, who died within weeks of her 100th birthday, hosted *Saturday Night Live* at 88, and continued her career in film and television until age 95.

Welcome to the new world of SuperAging—the most important social revolution we have ever seen.

THE SUPERAGING REVOLUTION

Of course, we already know that people are living longer. Someone turning 65 today can look forward to at least another 15 years, maybe a lot more. So it's no longer remarkable seeing people live into their 80s, or even 90s. In fact, the fastest-growing age group in percentage terms is centenarians.

What's new and different—revolutionary, in fact—is *how* those "aging years" are being spent. And that comes from a whole new way of looking at what aging is in the first place, along with a radical new way of managing it: **SuperAging**.

The old way (literally) is what we call **DefaultAging**. It still dominates healthcare, economics, housing, business, and virtually every aspect of how our society is organized. It sees "old" as a condition that kicks in, almost abruptly, when you reach the traditional retirement age of 65. "Old" means

- You haven't got much time left (maybe 10–15 years).
- You have worsening physical and mental health, so you can't do much and society shouldn't expect much.
- The best you can do, in fact, is to minimize your suffering to achieve a relatively pain-free and dignified glide path to the finish line, which isn't far away.

There are no positives, nothing else that "getting older" can bring you once you hit "old."

But that was before the SuperAging revolution.

We didn't invent the term "SuperAging." It has appeared in some articles, on a few websites, and in a handful of book subtitles—usually books on how to live longer. In fact, "longevity" is usually what triggers the phrase: adding years to your life span, living longer than what might have been expected, or certainly, longer than previous generations were able to accomplish.

But we think longevity (and SuperAging) can mean—*should* mean—much more than that. It's a totally new way to view what aging actually is: not just mathematically more years, but *different* years, with dramatically different characteristics. Instead of a relatively short, painful period of decline, aging now becomes a dynamic, positive time of life. Instead of mere survival, there is growth, development, new possibilities, and achievements.

You get older without getting "old"!

And as you get older, you don't just keep living, you actively pursue new things: you learn, you grow, you experiment, you discover.

Julia "Hurricane" Hawkins didn't take up competitive racing until she was 80.

Sir Tom was already 99 when he thought about his garden laps to raise money.

Prince Philip had to cut back his busy schedule because of a back problem at 87, but then went on for almost another decade before he "retired."

Manfred Steiner started his journey to a physics PhD at the age of 70.

And as for Senator Grassley, imagine making a decision to run for another six-year term when you're already 89! He was nominated—he won—and his new term won't expire until he's 95.

Each of these people saw their future as a time of continuing activity and achievement, and not merely the defensive management of decline. That's why all of them exemplify SuperAging.

Are there physical and mental challenges? Obviously. SuperAgers do not disregard the realities of physical decline; if anything, they're even more motivated than DefaultAgers to learn about and apply every possible technique to mitigate these harmful factors. A magic diet? A new fitness program? There are already many books on these subjects, and SuperAgers are certainly buying them.

But SuperAgers go way beyond those topics. Sure, you want to live longer. And you want to know the latest ideas for achieving that. But it's precisely because you have a good chance of succeeding that you need the SuperAging mindset.

Think about it this way. If you hit 65, you may well be looking at another 30-plus years (certainly 20-plus years) of life. What are you going to do with that time? Even to pose the question immediately opens up a huge new agenda. Employment or retirement. Learning and discovery. New places to live. New relationships. New challenges and opportunities. New experiences you haven't had before.

Don't you want to approach life through this wider lens? Don't you want to see *all* the possibilities?

If so, this book is for you.

1

THE 7*A*'S OF SUPERAGING

Isn't it funny how the word "old" is baked right into every description of age? Five years *old*. Twenty-five years *old*. Sixty years *old*. Life is presented as a countdown. Is it any wonder DefaultAging has persisted for so long? After all, the math is the math, and the bigger the number, the closer you are to "the end." Right? What else is there to aspire to, except to get to that end point as gently and painlessly as possible?

But life doesn't have to be a countdown. Or, to put it another way, the countdown can be relegated to the sidelines, and other factors can become much more important.

Try this one simple mental trick: imagine bringing a whole lifetime of knowledge, experience, skills, talent, relationships, wisdom (and, let's face it, money) to two or three more decades ahead of you in which to leverage all those assets into an ongoing wonderful experience.

Do you need to stay healthy? Of course. Do you need to worry about diet and fitness and various medical conditions and risks? Absolutely. But should that be the main agenda? There's so much more! And if you're going to grab all those extras, if you're going to aspire to be a SuperAger, you'll want to start with sorting out what you bring to the party and what new information or skills you'll want to acquire.

We've identified seven critical pillars that, collectively, enable you to switch from the narrow DefaultAging mindset to the wider, infinitely more exciting SuperAging lens. We call them the seven *A*'s of SuperAging: Attitude, Awareness, Activity, Accomplishment, Autonomy, Attachment, and Avoidance (of certain negative factors).

All are interrelated. All are synergistic. Each is necessary and each reinforces the others, building a complete SuperAging program. With the seven *A*'s, you'll change from "manage the decline" to "accomplish so much more."

Each chapter deals with a different one of the *A*'s and includes recommendations for the practical application of the information and the tools to create a lifelong SuperAging program of your own.

You may be a DefaultAger now—not because you've done anything wrong but because it just kind of crept up on you, or it seems like that's the way things have to be. But you can be a SuperAger instead. Let's get started!

THE PILLARS OF SUPERAGING

ATTITUDE

Attitude is the underpinning of the entire SuperAging revolution. There is a growing body of scientific research that demonstrates how people who have a positive attitude actually live longer than those who don't. But this requires more—much more—than just a vague, feel-good notion of optimism in general. It's anchored in a firm belief in the consequences of that optimism; you're entering a period with many exciting new possibilities. Which in turn means that you believe (a) you still have time to do a lot and (b) there's a lot you want to do. The positive attitude, then, is attached to a concrete vision of an exciting future. Do you have such a vision already? Can you create it? Yes—we'll show you how. And then, armed with that vision, how do you keep it fresh and active? This chapter will give you strategies to put this foundational pillar to work for you.

AWARENESS

In the DefaultAging world, the only knowledge that really mattered for this stage of life was knowledge about health, which was in the hands of healthcare professionals. The DefaultAgers were more or less passive recipients of whatever information the pros had or were inclined to provide. It wasn't up to you to keep track of all the latest research and development. Your doctor would tell you what you needed to know. Same for your money— your bankers or financial planners would keep you (more or less) informed.

But in the world of SuperAging, knowledge is moving from the insider, or the pros, into the hands of the SuperAgers themselves, who are *active seekers and consumers* of information. SuperAgers are not content to be passive receivers of whatever the system provides; they look for more and are quite ready to seek multiple opinions.

But that immediately leads to two challenges.

First, as we will see, they are seeking that information and those expert opinions across a much wider range of topics. It's not just health and wellness; it's retirement and employment, independent living, finance, community, the leveraging of science and technology, and more.

Second, the advent of the internet simultaneously made that information more accessible and yet more confusing. There has been an explosion of information on all topics, not just aging. The internet has fueled a massive increase in channels of information and a corresponding perceived decrease in the credibility and authority of the once-untouchable "established" authorities (whether that be your family doctor or a network TV anchor).

If you aspire to be a SuperAger, the good news is that there's plenty of information on the topics that matter. But that's also the bad news! You face a complex jungle of content: websites, YouTube channels, apps, Google searches—every topic related to aging now carries a flood of information that seems to grow by the hour. The challenge is in translating all that into a manageable, concrete plan.

It's clear that Awareness now demands a set of skills. It's more than just being able to find a helpful book (or e-book) or discovering a useful podcast. It increasingly requires an organized, systematic approach to information-gathering, and it must also include some way of curating the informational torrent so it can be digested, evaluated, and applied, while at the same time being constantly updated. How do you do all that? You'll find out in the Awareness chapter.

ACTIVITY

Physical activity—whether it's applied to diet and nutrition or exercise—is a tool shared, in some respects, by both DefaultAgers and SuperAgers who need and want to keep fit, mentally and physically. Both groups have an interest in good habits of diet along with a fitness regime that makes sense. SuperAgers, however, are more ready to widen the scope of Activity, particularly when Activity can mean learning new skills or exploring new approaches to nutrition or fitness and, increasingly, to brain health. As with everything else they touch, SuperAgers are stretching the meaning of Activity, and in chapter 4, we'll explore what that involves in more detail.

ACCOMPLISHMENT

One of the classic benchmarks of DefaultAging is "retirement," which is supposed to happen more or less automatically at age 65. Not anymore! SuperAgers are blowing up the whole notion of retiring at 65—or at all. Now we have full retirement, hybrid retirement, partial employment, home-based businesses, side gigs, and a dizzying array of permutations and combinations all leading to the same bottom line: SuperAgers want to keep on accomplishing things.

The most dramatic statistics are in the workplace, and we'll explore them fully, but it's a mistake to see this as only a matter of working versus retirement. There's also a rich menu of personal development and accomplishment, whether volunteering, mentoring, learning a new skill for no other reason than personal enrichment, or seeing Accomplishment as an opportunity to change or deepen relationships, such as through grandparenting, which offers a whole category of new approaches and creativity.

One of the big reasons why Accomplishment is such a key factor in SuperAging is that, by definition, Accomplishment implies having goals and plans to achieve them, which means having a sense of purpose, which in turn reinforces the first key item in the tool kit, Attitude.

AUTONOMY

SuperAgers want to have autonomy, ideally for the remainder of their lives.

It didn't take the COVID pandemic and a scandalously high number of fatalities occurring in nursing homes to make older people want to avoid ending their life in such an institution. The desire to stay at home for as long as possible, to "age in place," was already well established before COVID. And it's only getting stronger, fueled by exciting new developments in technology, from robots to AI that can transform your home itself into a caregiver. So if autonomy starts with where you live, there is a dazzling new menu of possibilities—but you have to know about them to be able to take advantage. (Awareness, again! See how all the tools are interconnected?)

But physical autonomy isn't the only challenge. There is also financial autonomy. Never before in history have we had to worry about the possibility of "outliving our money," but it's now a reality, thanks to longevity. Are there new investment strategies you need to know about? New ways of producing income? New systems (even apps) for controlling spending more effectively? Yes, yes, and yes. SuperAgers need, and welcome, all possible resources that can help them retain their autonomy while they are enjoying all the fruits of SuperAging.

ATTACHMENT

Many research studies have confirmed that isolation and loneliness among older people exerts a seriously harmful effect on health—and life span. Both DefaultAgers and SuperAgers are aware of this risk and motivated to do something about it. But SuperAgers are much more likely to expand the range of tools and techniques they deploy.

The first level of Attachment is, of course, the immediate family. Both DefaultAgers and SuperAgers alike face a wide range of situations—close-knit families, families who are geographically close but not particularly connected otherwise, families who are geographically far apart but emotionally close, families who have drifted apart both physically and operationally. There is also a wide range of family contributions to health and well-being, from social and emotional support all the way to intensive physical caregiving. At the most basic level, there may not be much of a divide between how DefaultAgers and SuperAgers respond to their family situation and try to maximize the benefits of family relationships.

The difference is that DefaultAgers are more likely to stop with maintaining and protecting their existing relationships while SuperAgers are more likely to reach for more. They're much more likely to use digital tools, for example, to go beyond immediate family and create online relationships that reduce social isolation. And it isn't just a matter of one-to-one digital encounters. There are also exciting ideas about new kinds of housing and communities that can foster much richer and more dynamic relationships and experiences. A hot new concept, for example, is the location of housing facilities for seniors, rich in amenities, right on the campuses of universities, creating exciting new intergenerational possibilities.

In the Attachment chapter, you'll read the latest ideas and see how SuperAgers are using them.

AVOIDANCE

All the pillars presented so far are positive and proactive, producing important results. The final one goes the other way: it identifies negative forces that SuperAgers will want to avoid (or, being SuperAgers, actively challenge and combat).

The most important is *ageism*, which can take the form of blatant discrimination (especially in the workforce) or much more subtly through patronization or condescension, particularly from professionals like doctors or financial advisers who still have outmoded views of what aging is and are apt to stereotype you as being much less capable than you really are. (We call it the "there, there, dear" syndrome.)

Ageism permeates our environment: most politicians (even 80-something representatives and senators) and certainly almost all policy makers are at least 10–15 years behind the times in their understanding of what is going on among the older age cohorts. Marketers and their ad agencies have also been slow to fully appreciate the breathtaking consumer spending opportunities they have thanks to longevity, and so they continue to prioritize and pursue younger age groups, notably the Millennials who can't yet contribute the spending power the marketers require. There is no good reason for SuperAgers to accept these negative forces, and we'll show you how to take action against them.

Action is needed, too, to keep up with the nonstop barrage of frauds and scams that target older people. Here again, there is a strong menu of resources that can help, and we'll explore them.

A WIDE-ANGLE APPROACH

Embracing all seven pillars is your best path to SuperAging. But if we look at all seven pillars of SuperAging and the associated tools and techniques for applying them, we can see that the first two—Attitude and Awareness—are necessary conditions for properly using the remaining five. Each of those deal with a more specific issue (health and wellness, career and retirement, self-determination, social connectivity, and circumventing negative forces). So each involves distinct needs and requires skills of its own. But without the necessary Attitude or an efficient system for maintaining Awareness, you won't be able to fully explore the other issues and utilize the other tools.

Here's how the elements are interrelated:

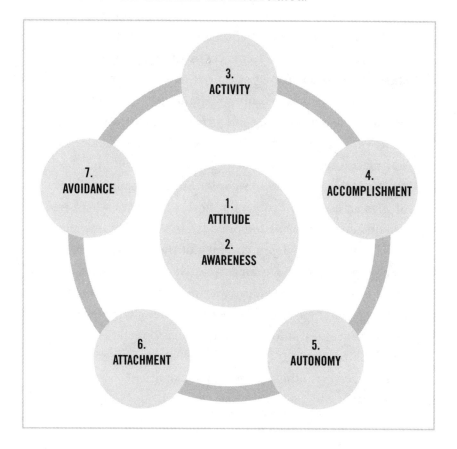

What will shift you into a SuperAger is the intelligent—and consistent—attention to *all* the A's. By broadening your agenda, you set yourself up to really maximize the potential of what could easily be 20 or 30 years (or more) of life span after the age of 65. This is how you "get older without getting old," how you live with purpose and energy and fulfillment.

Don't Forget the Companion Website, SuperAging.info!

As you'll see when you read the coming chapters, the SuperAging topic is jam-packed with information—maybe too much information, which is why we think you need this book as a curator of what really matters and what to do about it. But you also need to recognize that the information isn't static. There is a constant stream of new discoveries in science, products, and resources; "the longevity business" is not only real but booming and growing, and we wouldn't be doing you a service if we didn't also provide a mechanism for staying current and updated.

That's the role of our website, SuperAging.info. Think of it as an essential companion to this book. It's where we will update the information provided in these chapters, plus bring you more in-depth coverage of the topics, including videos, podcasts, and even interactive surveys where you can express your own ideas and meet other like-minded SuperAgers. There will also be a free e-newsletter that will bring the freshest information and ideas directly into your email inbox.

Be sure to visit the website and bookmark it!

2

ATTITUDE

Having a positive attitude is widely, and almost automatically, seen as a Good Thing. It's certainly a staple of self-help books and other programs, with a pedigree going back almost a century.

- In 1936, Dale Carnegie produced the book *How to Win Friends and Influence People*, which went on to sell over 30 million copies worldwide. The basic strategy: a positive mental attitude.
- A year later, Napoleon Hill wrote *Think and Grow Rich*, which purported to give the money-making "secrets" of millionaires like Andrew Carnegie and Thomas Edison. The secrets all came down to being positive—so positive you could actually *see* the money you were going to make.
- Fifteen years later, in 1952, Norman Vincent Peale published *The Power of Positive Thinking*, which sold more than five million copies worldwide. "Picture yourself succeeding," Peale advised. "Think a positive thought to drown out a negative thought."

The extensions of this foundational idea are widespread, touching virtually every aspect of life. Successful sports teams have a "winning attitude." Salespeople are trained to shrug off rejection and "stay positive." Having a positive mental attitude has even been branded with an enormous array of retreats, seminars, and at-home training programs carried out by coaches, practitioners, commentators, and other (real or self-proclaimed) experts.

In sum, everyone agrees: Attitude matters, and obviously it's better to be positive than negative.

The trouble is, the idea can seem kind of squishy. Though it makes a rough intuitive sense, is it backed up by hard evidence? Is there some kind of observable *mechanism* that enables Attitude to achieve the outcomes claimed for it?

The answer is yes. We can show you proof of a direct link between attitude and longevity. There are even some scientific measurements that, for the first time, suggest *how* and *why* a positive attitude works to produce these outcomes.

But where does a positive attitude come from? Is it something you either have or don't have? Can it be acquired? Or made even stronger if you already have it? Let's find out.

DO OPTIMISTS REALLY LIVE LONGER?

There is now strong, research-based evidence that, yes, a positive mental attitude contributes directly to a longer life span. Here are just a few sources that dig into this.

In a study involving 70,000 people who were followed for 10 to 30 years, researchers at Boston University School of Medicine found that optimistic people can live up to 15% longer than pessimistic people.

Another study published in *Psychological Science* looked at data from over 6,000 participants who were asked to agree or disagree with statements about having a purpose in life. (For example, "Some people wander aimlessly through life, but I am not one of them.") The respondents were followed for 14 years. By the end, about 9% of the sample had died. Those who had died had reported a lower purpose in life than the survivors.

Being more optimistic as you age is one thing, but how about using positive mental attitude to "think yourself young"? That's the provocative question asked in an article in the *Guardian*, which surveyed several pieces of research to arrive at the startling conclusion that those who "see the ageing process as a potential for personal growth" are more likely to have better health in their 70s through 90s than those who consider aging to be about helplessness and decline. In one study, people in their 70s and 80s who briefly imagined themselves to still be younger outscored a control group on a battery of physical and cognitive tests. Some who had arthritis even saw reductions in inflammation.

Or consider this study from the Yale School of Public Health, which started in 1975 with 1,000 subjects having an average age of 63. They were asked to agree or disagree with statements about aging. (For example, "As you get older, you are less useful.") They were then followed and their health outcomes were tracked for almost 30 years, until 2002. The average person with a positive attitude lived on for just over 22 years after the start, while those with more negative attitudes to aging lived on only 15 years. In other words, the optimists had almost a 50% higher remaining life span than the pessimists.

THE MIND-BODY CONNECTION OF POSITIVITY

If having a positive mental attitude is strongly associated with living longer, the next question is: Why? How does it work? The proof is in these studies, which show science-backed evidence that there is some mechanism, some measurably positive physical effect on the body, produced by feelings of optimism or a sense of purpose.

A 2019 paper published in the *Journal of the American Medical Association* studied nearly 7,000 adults over the age of 50 and found that those who scored highest on a scale that measured purpose in life were less likely to die during the four-year study period than those with lower scores. Why? Having a stronger purpose in life was associated with decreased expression of pro-inflammatory genes. Another study found that strong purpose may be associated with the regulation of stress hormones by enabling accelerated stress recovery.

The *Guardian* article mentioned earlier also pointed out that elderly people with negative attitudes or expectations about aging have higher systolic blood pressure when responding to challenges, while those with positive ideas tend to respond to challenges with less stress. For the pessimists, bodily inflammation rises; for the optimists, much less so.

There's even some evidence of impact at the individual cellular level. Each of our chromosomes has protective caps called telomeres that keep the DNA from being damaged. As we age, these telomeres shorten, and there is a ton of interesting research going on right now aimed at preventing this shortening from happening, or even reversing it. But another factor may influence this mechanism. It appears that the telomere-shortening process is accelerated among people with negative attitudes and slower among the optimists. So even before any new research or therapies kick in, the optimists appear to be making positive things happen at the cellular level.

A 2017 article by AARP reported on a study by Cornell University and Weill Cornell Medical College. Researchers asked 175 participants, with ages ranging from 40 to 65, to report their positive emotions for 30 days. Researchers then collected blood samples and analyzed them for three biomarkers of inflammation. Result: A greater diversity of day-to-day positive emotions correlated with lower systemic inflammation. But it really only worked if there was a wide range of positive feelings. In fact, the researchers coined the term "emodiversity" to mean a "breadth and abundance" of positive emotions, including being active, alert, amused, at ease, attentive, calm, cheerful, determined, enthusiastic, excited, happy, inspired, interested, proud, relaxed, and strong. Yes, 16 in all, and the more of them you possess every day, the better.

It's also been demonstrated that a positive attitude contributes to faster recovery from illness or medical procedures, which in turn plays into longevity. In this context, a 2018 study reported in *Newsweek* found that religious people live four years longer than average.

These studies are just the tip of the iceberg. Positive attitude, feeling of optimism, sense of purpose—there is overwhelming, measurable evidence that these emotions are correlated with a longer and healthier life.

FAITH AND SPIRITUALITY

An important subset of positive attitude is faith, whether formal religious belief or simply a feeling of spirituality or connectedness to something higher or outside the physical bounds of body and environment, and also often accompanied by active techniques such as meditation.

There is statistical evidence showing that people of faith live longer. Is it the faith itself—i.e., the specific beliefs—or merely the positive effects of being part of a community? (We'll explore this further in the chapter on Activity.) The important point is that the topic has been looked at closely, and the statistical correlation between faith and longevity seems very strong.

NATURE OR NURTURE?

The next logical question is: Where does this positive attitude come from? Is it just a part of your personality that you are born with or do you develop it without really noticing?

The science is split. For many years, the prevailing wisdom was that more people were, by nature, optimistic than pessimistic. For example, a 2009 study of more than 150,000 adults from 140 countries found that 89% of respondents had an optimistic expectation for the world over the next five years, and 95% were optimistic about their own futures. According to another study analyzing 500 pairs of twins, half of them reared together and half of them adopted apart early in life, about 25% of optimism could be attributed to genes.

In addition, an optimistic outlook is encouraged socially at a young age and may then be adopted simply as a rational means of gaining favor. Research shows that children as young as preschoolers prefer hanging with kids who have a cheery attitude over a negative one. In order to be accepted, then, it would make sense to be that kind of child. So, long before a preschooler even hears or understands the actual word "optimism," there may be a strong influence in that direction.

That finding has been challenged, however. Other studies

suggest we are "wired for pessimism." But there may be a healthy reason: pessimism can make us more realistic about the outside world and prevent us from falling into delusional traps where we may overestimate the chances for a sunny outcome and wind up paying a harmful price for our misjudgment.

Is it better to expect the worst and be pleasantly surprised? One study out of Denmark was interesting: it reported that Danes consistently score higher on life-satisfaction questions than any other Western country. Was it hair color? ("Blondes have more fun!") Genes? Food? Climate? The authors reviewed all these factors but then proposed a more provocative reason. Danes are pessimists, always expecting the worst. Then they're pleased when things turn out to be not quite as bad.

The bottom line seems to be that the presence of optimism or pessimism, whatever any genetic predisposition, is still heavily dependent on experience and learning. You see situations, you form judgments (positive or negative) about likely outcomes, events prove you right or wrong, and you adapt your attitudes accordingly. These accumulate and coalesce into an attitudinal underpinning that tilts toward optimism or pessimism.

But that underpinning is constantly being applied to new situations and new circumstances. What has happened to us so far? What do we think is going to happen in relation to the new factor or situation that we are evaluating?

This process is exactly what happens to your ideas about, and response to, aging. You bring with you some mix of positive and negative based on a combination of your nature plus your learnings and experiences with other topics. You then apply these to new information and observations. The process is dynamic, not static. You may start out pessimistic about the prospects of aging and then be won over by the evidence you see around you. That's certainly our objective here.

THE TWO CORE FOUNDATIONS OF THE SUPERAGING ATTITUDE

Let's set aside that 25% genetic factor that may go into optimism or pessimism and look at learning and experience. When it comes to aging, there are two key factors that become the foundations of the SuperAging attitude:

1. **Longevity.** What's the current state of play? How long can we live? What is objectively realistic?
2. **Who is doing the aging?** What has our life experience been so far? What are our accumulated learnings, attitudes, and responses to other challenges and opportunities?

LONGEVITY

Both DefaultAging and SuperAging are based on a model of how we age, how long we can live, and what is expected to happen at various ages along the timeline. We've developed two schematics to illustrate the models. Both are evidence-driven responses to what can be clearly seen—then and now—in the outside world.

If you're a DefaultAger, you aren't doing anything wrong, and you haven't deliberately decided to reject the idea of living longer and doing much more with those extra years. It's just that you are holding on to a model of aging that is now obsolete. Let's look at that model more closely.

THE DEFAULTAGING TIMELINE

Up until the last decade or so, the DefaultAging model prevailed because it was actually true. And it had been true for over a century. The human life span had distinct phases with an age range attached to each. Regardless of an individual's attitudinal predisposition (optimist or pessimist), there was really no choice but to accept the reality of the model.

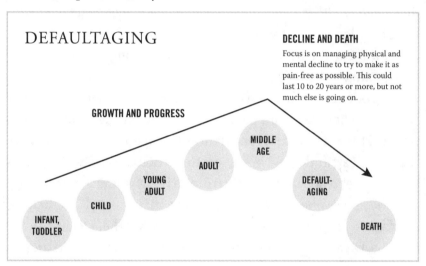

DEFAULTAGING

DECLINE AND DEATH
Focus is on managing physical and mental decline to try to make it as pain-free as possible. This could last 10 to 20 years or more, but not much else is going on.

GROWTH AND PROGRESS

MIDDLE AGE

ADULT

YOUNG ADULT

DEFAULT-AGING

CHILD

INFANT, TODDLER

DEATH

As you can see, life has two big stages: Growth and Progress, followed by Decline and Death. Growth and Progress takes you from birth to retirement (at age 65); Decline and Death is what happens for the remainder of your life.

The model makes it clear that the Decline and Death stage is short, usually no more than a decade or so. This was true right up through the 1990s; the average 65-year-old had about 10 to 12 more years of life expectancy. Given so few years—compared to the six decades you spent getting there—it's obvious that there was little point in making any dramatic new plans. There simply weren't enough years left to "reinvent" yourself, to seriously pursue a new career or new interests, or to look on this period as one of new opportunity, discovery, or growth.

The best you could aspire to was a reasonably gentle glide path to the finish. You hoped to get through it with a minimum of pain and suffering. You might even be happy during these years. Retirement was often presented, especially in advertising, as a time when you could finally relax and enjoy doing nothing. It wasn't necessarily bad. But it was, by definition, extremely limited. Sure, there might be some outliers here and there who lived a lot longer, kept working past the age of 65, or took up new activities. For the overwhelming majority, though, DefaultAging was, in effect, the only game in town.

It produced a collection of perceptions and beliefs about what was to be expected from people when they hit the DefaultAging phase. This was no different than other age-related stereotypes that linked attitudes and behaviors to particular phases along life's timeline (rebellious teens, upwardly striving young adults, empty nesters). Everyone—academics, policy makers and politicians, marketers—applied these characteristics to the DefaultAgers, and the DefaultAgers obligingly applied these characteristics to themselves:

- Retirement: a disengagement from the working world and, gradually, from the social world.
- A drastic curtailment in spending: Older consumers were of little or no interest to marketers, who wrote them off as a group whose brand habits were long ago frozen in stone (so why chase after them with advertising?) and that wasn't going to be around long enough to spend much more in the future anyway. This was the accepted wisdom in virtually every product category, from cars to packaged goods to fashion.

- The end of romance and a sex life.
- A steady physical and quite possibly mental decline (from conditions such as dementia and Alzheimer's).
- Little or no further meaningful additions to life's résumé, such as new ambitions or accomplishments.

This is how society saw the age group, and this is how the age group saw itself. There wasn't much time left, and therefore not much reason to view the final phase with any real zest.

But today there is a new reality. And just as DefaultAging and its mindset was a function of how aging actually worked at that time, SuperAging is a response to a new reality, a dramatic change in the model driven by one key force: *longevity*.

THE SUPERAGING TIMELINE

The reality of dramatically longer life spans is destroying the DefaultAging model. Here is what the new reality looks like:

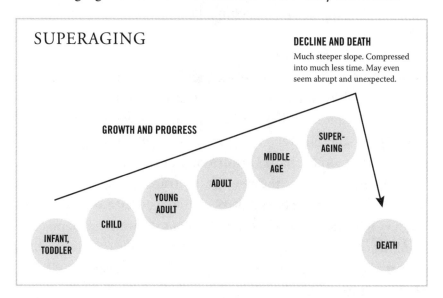

In this model, the Decline and Death stage does not kick in at age 65. Rather, there is a long period of continued health and activity, which we have dubbed the SuperAging phase. It belongs with the Growth and Progress part of life. The Decline and Death phase eventually comes, of course, but it comes much later, and is much shorter with a steeper trajectory. You could make it into your 90s as a SuperAger, and then have one really bad year where everything collapses and concludes with your death. In fact, you could make it to 100 or more before this happens.

As this model becomes increasingly real and achievable, the DefaultAging timeline is destroyed and the SuperAging timeline takes over. Even if, for the sake of the exercise, we kept 65 as the same jumping-off point for what comes after middle age, we're now looking at a very possible scenario of 25 SuperAging years, perhaps even more. So it makes no sense to treat those years as if they had nothing else to offer but warding off age-related pain and mitigating decline. Now you *do* have time to make new plans, set new goals, accomplish new things.

Longevity, then, is the primary driver of SuperAging because longevity has increasingly become the reality of what comes after middle age.

It shouldn't be surprising that this new reality is the foundation of SuperAging. Not "positive attitude" in a vacuum or because of predispositions, but as a product of observation, a response to what can be seen happening in the real world. SuperAgers understand and embrace the totally different landscape of what aging has become, thanks to dramatic extensions in life span. This understanding of the new reality transcends the variations in their individual personalities. Obviously, not every one of them will by nature be a Norman Vincent Peale model of positive thinking. But it doesn't matter; it's understanding the radical changes in what aging has become that turns every intelligent observer into a SuperAger.

This doesn't mean that personal characteristics or predispositions have nothing to do with the matter, however. While SuperAging would be impossible without the reality of longevity, it is also accelerated by the attitudinal characteristics of the generations who are actually doing the aging.

WHO IS DOING THE AGING?

If the main question is "What has life span become?" then close behind are more questions: "*Who* is doing the aging? What do they already bring to the party?"

This leads us, unavoidably, to a comparison of the various generations who are involved. At the moment, three generations are engaged with DefaultAging versus SuperAging:

- The Greatest Generation, born between 1910 and 1929
- The Silent Generation, born between 1930 and 1944
- The Baby Boomers, born between 1945 and 1964

Let's look at the major events and influences on each generation, and the major attitudes and behavioral traits they display.

Major life events and influences:

- Greatest Generation
  - Great Depression
  - World War II
- Silent Generation
  - World War II
  - Postwar boom

- Cold War
- Space race
- Start of civil rights movement
- Baby Boomers
  - Postwar boom
  - Vietnam War
  - Civil rights struggle
  - Social radicalism (sex, drugs) followed by materialism (Yuppies)

Major attitudes and behavioral traits:

- Greatest Generation
  - High sense of responsibility, sense of duty, patriotism
  - Money savers, not spenders
- Silent Generation
  - Best educated to date
  - Disciplined, successful
  - Younger half (born 1939 on) share many attributes with Boomers
- Baby Boomer Generation
  - Huge population = considerable influence in society, marketplace
  - Often seen as selfish ("Me" generation)
  - Intense work ethic
  - Risk-takers, trendsetters

- Note: The nicknames assigned to each generation are widely used in demographic reports, marketing analyses, and social science literature. The dates of birth are not set in stone; different demographers posit slightly different starting and ending points, but the numbers presented here are widely accepted, and a fluctuation of a year or two doesn't materially change the picture.

We have to accept, up front, that generational comparisons like this can never be precisely accurate (or completely fair). Obviously not every single Baby Boomer is exactly the same. That said, there is a wealth of behavioral research to demonstrate that it is possible to identify certain attitudes and behaviors that predominate within a particular generation, compared to another generation, and that arise from the unique circumstances and life experiences of that generation.

The Greatest Generation was so called (most importantly by Tom Brokaw, who wrote a bestseller with that title) because they lived through the Great Depression as children and adolescents, and then showed up uncomplainingly to fight in World War II. For them, DefaultAging was the dominant reality. They did not drive (nor could they reasonably have been expected to drive) SuperAging.

Things start to get more interesting with the Silent Generation, so called because they were seen to have cashed in on the postwar economic boom and became the stereotypical suburbanites, the comfortable "Eisenhower Republicans"— complacent, obedient, disciplined. Yet the younger tranche— born between the late 1930s and 1944, let's say—displayed attitudes and behaviors that more closely resembled the Baby Boomers who followed immediately behind them. They were more likely to question authority, not just with the ritual juvenile rebelliousness that has characterized every generation in history, but with concrete activities that deliberately sought to disrupt and bring about change. The leaders of the then-revolutionary Free Speech Movement at Berkeley or the Students for a Democratic Society, the people who stood shoulder to shoulder with Martin

Luther King Jr. and the Freedom Riders, and the activists of the movement against the Vietnam War were all born in the last five years or so of the Silent Generation.

Then came the Boomers, with more of the same. Ready to upset all the norms. Hyperactive, goal-oriented, and concerned (some would say obsessively concerned) with achievement. And always the center of attention! Because of their sheer numbers, they've had the spotlight on themselves at every single age they've passed through (especially as the prime target of advertisers). Why should they now accept the passivity of DefaultAging? Why should they agree to step offstage and out of the spotlight?

Thus we have, in attitudinal terms, the trailing chunk of the Silent Generation plus the entire Baby Boomer generation—a massive number of people (over 90 million in the United States alone) who are accustomed to being disruptive and driving change.

And it's not just external change like reforming society, but internal change like redefining one's self. The Boomers, after all, morphed from the hippies of Woodstock to the Yuppies of Wall Street without batting an eye. So in sum, we have here some important *generational predispositions* that also contribute to the SuperAging revolution.

We can prove this with a simple thought experiment. Take a look at the photos below and then, using what you know about the younger Silent Generation members plus all the Baby Boomers, answer the question.

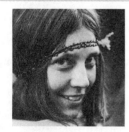
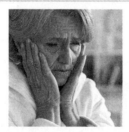
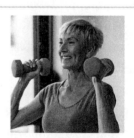

Did *she* age into . . .   . . . her?   . . . or her?

The left-hand photo represents an attendee at the legendary Woodstock festival, in the summer of 1969. Let's assume the young lady was born right at the start of Baby Boomer–hood, in 1945. So she would have been 24 back then, and 76 years old today. Which version of "76 years old" do you think she aspired to?

The question answers itself, doesn't it?

We can provide solid evidence too, and not just an instinctual feeling that the more positive direction is the way things have gone.

It started, even before the possibility of radical longevity really kicked in, with a rebellion against the word "senior." As far back as 2002, there was an article (by Susan J. Ellis on energizeinc .com) titled "Don't Call Me a 'Senior'!" that anticipated the continued extension of life span and pointed out how "one could be considered a 'senior' for fully half of one's lifetime!" Five years later, Jack Rosenthal pointed out in the *New York Times* that "no variation of *elderly*" could cover the "vast variety and abilities" of those older than 55 or 65. He noted, correctly, that "oldsters" or "golden agers" were patronizing terms, and that "senior" might be acceptable as an adjective (as in senior vice president), but not as a noun, to identify a group.

We can see, then, a cultural pushback against DefaultAging even before the full scope and potential of longevity was a reality. Its advent was sensed, certainly, and there were many signs of where it might lead, but in 2007 it was still rational for a 65-year-old to believe that they had, at best, 10 to 15 years to go and that the dominant issue was still to reduce age-related pain and suffering and hope for a relatively gentle glide to the not-too-distant finish line. Refuse to retire "automatically" at 65? Shoot for a PhD when you're already 70? Take up competitive sprinting at 80? Not yet in sight.

Even so, the underlying attitudes, the pushback against the stereotypes that had defined aging throughout human history, were already in place, and searching for new terms of reference.

Let's take a look at some other prominent signs. As you read all these examples, recall our little thought experiment with the young lady from Woodstock. It's not that hard to imagine her rejecting her grandmother's vision of aging and preferring that of Jane Juska.

SKIING

By 2008 (when David's first book, *The New Old*, appeared) many Baby Boomers were proudly proclaiming their unwillingness to sacrifice any further for the sake of their children (as previous generations, most notably the Greatest Generation, had certainly done). SKIing became a Thing. It stands for "spending the kids' inheritance," and it was openly declared on bumper stickers and T-shirts.

There were even books that could show you how to do it. British TV star Annie Hulley, who had also made a fortune in real estate, was one author who offered specific advice in her book titled *How to Spend the Kids' Inheritance*. Lest it be thought that this was just an exercise in frivolous good fun, Hulley offers a serious rationale that includes what is already true of longevity. She points out that our ancestors lived shorter lives and now it's becoming obvious that a life of "toil today with the hope of rest tomorrow" isn't realistic anymore. According to her, with people living longer, "you might have to 'Spend the Kids' Inheritance' (SKI)" to make ends meet.

This last point is huge. It speaks to the possibility of actually outliving your money, an idea that never existed before the longevity that powers SuperAging. We'll have a lot more to say about it in the chapter on Autonomy. For now, let's just note that it is another powerful underpinning to SuperAging. The ability to keep going and not automatically retire may be not only physically and emotionally desirable but also financially necessary.

SEX

Around that same time, "sex for seniors" became a topic. In 2006, author Gail Sheehy, who had begun tracking women through their life stages in her 1976 bestseller, *Passages*, brought out *Sex and the Seasoned Woman*. Hundreds of Baby Boomer women (and those older) talked to her candidly about their sex lives. "A seasoned woman is spicy," she wrote. "She has been marinated in life experience." Sheehy goes on to explain that older women are less likely to have an agenda, since they no longer have a biological clock to consider, and tend to be playful, confident, and secure in who they are.

Three years earlier, a retired California teacher named Jane Juska had published *A Round-Heeled Woman*, which reported on an experiment she had undertaken beginning in 1999, when she was 66. She ran a classified ad in the *New York Times Book Review* stating that, before she hit 67, she wanted to have a great deal of sex with someone she liked, adding, "If you want to talk first, Trollope works for me." Flooded with responses, she carefully chose a few, flew to New York, and had enough action to fill not only her first book but a follow-up called *Unaccompanied Women*. "The best sex I had," she said in an interview (with David's wife, Cynthia), "was with a man I was not in love with but whom I liked enormously, and with a man I adored but who was 32 so love was out of the question, or so I thought."

In 2007, research published in the *New England Journal of Medicine* based on interviews with over 3,000 men and women aged 57 to 85 showed a surprisingly high degree of sexual activity at all ages; limitations seemed to be driven more by health problems or lack of a partner rather than age. Sex with a partner in the previous year was reported by 73% of those aged 57 to 64, 53% of those aged 64 to 75, and 23% of those aged 75 to 85.

There's certainly been no slowdown. A 2019 survey by Lumen,

a dating app for singles over 50, interviewed 2,000 sexually active people aged 50 to 80 in the United States. Over 60% were still having sex, and almost a quarter (22%) said their sex lives were as adventurous as when they were younger.

In that same vein, in April 2022, an article on BBC.com says it all: "Are Baby Boomers Having the Best Time in Bed?" The answer is right in the subhead: "Older adults are often passed over in conversations about intimacy. But they may be having more fun than everyone else." (They're also contracting STDs at a high rate, as shown by the 164% jump in the number of cases of gonorrhea among Americans aged 55 and older between 2014 and 2018.)

ONLINE DATING

Online dating for seniors emerged at this same time. Major dating websites of that era, like Lavalife, spun off seniors' sections (or separate websites entirely, under different brand names). And there were the cougars—women who were pursuing younger men specifically for sex. Not surprisingly, they created websites where they could display their attributes. The trend is still alive today.

GRAY DIVORCE

Older adults were also ready to jettison relationships that were no longer working (we'll have much more on this in the chapter on Attachment). The so-called gray divorce phenomenon has seen divorce rates after age 50 double between 1990 and 2015. Wherever you look, the Boomers continue to push against previous norms and expectations.

THE SPECIFIC ATTITUDES THAT DRIVE SUPERAGING

Let's now briefly itemize the specific attitudes that spring from these foundations, and that make up the SuperAgers' Attitude toward the future.

"I HAVE TIME TO MAKE SERIOUS AND SATISFYING PLANS."

SuperAgers are optimistic because they believe there are solid grounds for that optimism. While many of them use digital apps to help them predict just how many years they may have left, even without that specificity they believe they have enough years left to set worthwhile goals and make plans.

The "bucket list" phenomenon is one good indicator of this attitude. (The movie came out in 2007, which shows again that the attitude was making itself felt even before the most dramatic increases in longevity.) By definition, if you have a bucket list—things you want to do before you die—you have at least some foundational belief in the possibility of checking off many, if not all, of the items. Another strong indicator is the emergence of lifestyle and reinvention coaches. Boomers are hiring consultants to help them scope out and plan the next phases of life. In the Accomplishment chapter we'll meet two of them.

A third strong indicator is that the "enough time left" concept is being endorsed by numerous experts who are themselves tearing up previous models of longevity, along with the expectations that flow from those models. In March 2022, J.P. Morgan Asset Management updated their guidelines to plan on having their clients live to 100 (more on this in the chapter on

Autonomy). So it's not just the Boomers who are latching on to this idea on their own; they're seeing it everywhere and having it reinforced from all directions.

"I WANT TO CONTINUE MY PERSONAL DEVELOPMENT."

Every early phase of life, even in the DefaultAging model, was characterized by growth and development. From basic childhood skills to lessons in independence as a teen, to the acquisition of professional credentials as a young adult, to parenting skills, and career development and financial strength, you could look back at every stage and say, "This is how I grew. This is what I learned. This is how I progressed." But then, suddenly, it stopped. You hit "old age" and there was nothing more. You were on that glide path we talked about, that 10-, 12-, at best 15-year off-ramp from life to death, where the only question was how painful and debilitating it would be. But further personal development? New learning? New skills? New experiences? Forget it. Not enough time. And besides, you were defined as "old"—meaning frail, weak, maybe totally helpless, just treading water until the end.

But not anymore. Not with SuperAging. Now, that final period is seen as one with just as much promise as the previous phases. True, the details will be different, and while the reality of physical and mental decline can't be ignored, the idea that this is an empty period is firmly rejected. SuperAgers see no reason why they can't continue to grow and develop, to learn new things, and to benefit from new experiences.

For instance, a growing number of Baby Boomers are going back to school, and the academic community is providing plenty of opportunity. Many universities that are struggling with declining enrollments are starting to see the "older" market as just that—a market, and a potentially important one. The Osher Lifelong Learning Institute, to take just one example, provides noncredit, nongraded courses for adults 50 and up, at over 120 colleges and universities across the United States.

Success stories are many, and SuperAgers are always in the headlines as they obtain degrees at ages that would have seemed impossible in earlier generations. In 2021, Varathaledchumy Shanmuganathan, an 87-year-old grandmother from Sri Lanka, became the oldest student to receive a master's degree from York University. Colette Bourlier earned a PhD at the age of 91, defending a thesis she had begun 30 years earlier at the University of Franche-Comté in Besançon, in eastern France. Pat Ormond, 75, and her granddaughter, Melody, both received degrees on the same day from the University of Tennessee at Chattanooga. What was interesting here is that Pat was a retired bookkeeper, but her degree was in anthropology with a major in archaeology. These examples all prove that it is never too late to continue personal development.

"I WANT TO KEEP WORKING."

With DefaultAging, the word "retirement" had a very precise meaning. You worked full-time for 40 years or so, and you accumulated enough (savings, pension, or other assets) so that you could stop working altogether and "enjoy" your remaining years in some measure of peace and dignity. Your working life, therefore, had an on switch (full-time employment) and an off switch (no employment at all), and the switch was thrown at age 65.

With SuperAging, that rigid either/or construct is completely gone.

Many SuperAgers want to keep working because it provides

many benefits to health and well-being (more on this in the chapter on Autonomy). Many others want to keep working because, well, they *need* to keep working; they don't have enough money saved up to fund their remaining years. This is not particularly surprising. The DefaultAging model only provides funds to support, on average, a dozen retirement years. Now, with longevity, those same funds (assuming retirement at 65) might have to carry you for twice as long. Can it be done? Hint: not likely.

The solutions vary widely: partial retirement, new career altogether, part-time employment, side hustle, acquisition of a small (particularly home-based) business. And even for those who fully retire, as per the DefaultAging model, "work" has been redefined through other avenues like volunteering, mentoring, and social engagement.

"I WANT TO KEEP ON BEING INFLUENTIAL."

If there was one thing the late-stage Silent Generation (and even more so, the Baby Boomers) were sure about, it was that they *mattered*. From childhood to middle age, they were eagerly sought out—by marketers, politicians, and opinion makers. If they weren't, as a generation, already on center stage, they knew how to elbow themselves into the spotlight. They marched, they demonstrated, they voted, they spent their dollars or withheld their spending. For better or worse, they called the shots.

Why should they stop now?

To such a population, the DefaultAging model is distasteful. Now you're "old." You're already weaker, and you're heading for utter helplessness. Where you were once independent, now you're relying on the kindness and consideration of younger people who are often (without malice) very patronizing and condescending. (Nothing drives Baby Boomers crazier than being condescended to; "there, there, dear," remember?)

This was bad enough when there wasn't much you could do about it—i.e., when the dramatic advances toward radical longevity hadn't really kicked in yet. Now that those advances are becoming real, now that it's plausible to aspire to *decades* of life after age 65, the surrender and the loss of influence built into the DefaultAging model have become intolerable. SuperAgers just won't act that way. They believe not only that they can continue to have active, engaged lives, but that those lives matter to society and to the future.

"IF I STAY ON TOP OF THINGS, I CAN LIVE A LOT LONGER."

SuperAgers extend their attitude and predisposition toward being *active* all the way into the business of being a SuperAger itself. They see it as something that doesn't fall into their lap, no matter how much optimism and energy they bring. It's something that requires work, knowledge (much more on this in the next chapter), careful thought, and the proactive seeking out of whatever can help.

The best example is healthcare.

DefaultAgers certainly cared about their health and were happy to receive help in the form of information or new drugs or therapies. But they were essentially passive recipients of whatever their doctors gave them. This passivity was reflected in their approach to the whole topic: They were *reactive*. They went to the doctor when they got sick, and then they didn't go again until the next time they got sick. And whatever the doctor said, it was received without question. The doctor was God.

SuperAgers, by contrast, are *proactive*. They seek out the information themselves, and the doctor, particularly if they are a general practitioner, is gradually morphing from God to Supplier. Doctors are rated on the internet today. There are online communities where patients with a common ailment can share ideas about what works and what doesn't. Google lets you price-compare virtually every procedure, including surgery. (The search term "discount heart surgery" produces about 25 million results!)

MAKE ATTITUDE PART OF YOUR SUPERAGING PROGRAM

Let's now look at how to apply all this to you. We said in the introduction that all the seven *A*'s of SuperAging are interconnected and mutually supportive. Nowhere is this truer than on the topic of Attitude. Whatever you brought with you before you started reading, be assured that a more positive outlook will be your rock-solid foundation in approaching all components of SuperAging.

So let's work on an Attitude adjustment, starting by understanding its two components:

- **Macro:** Your knowledge of and attitude toward aging.
- **Micro:** Your individual personality, and your optimist/pessimist balance.

Though these components work together, they are independent of each other. We'll measure both components with self-quizzes.

GAIN A MACRO OUTLOOK

Let's start with what you know or think about aging itself. We've designed a self-quiz that can serve as a convenient inventory of your perceptions. Below are a series of statements. For each one, please write down the number that comes closest to your current belief or feeling. Plan to repeat the quiz again after you've finished the book to see if your outlook has changed. For that reason, don't write your answers directly into the text, but on a separate sheet of paper, so that when you repeat the exercise you won't be influenced by how you answered the first time around.

- Choose 5 if you STRONGLY AGREE with the statement.
- Choose 4 if you SOMEWHAT AGREE with the statement.
- Choose 3 if you're neutral: you NEITHER AGREE NOR DISAGREE with the statement.
- Choose 2 if you SOMEWHAT DISAGREE with the statement.
- Choose 1 if you STRONGLY DISAGREE with the statement.

1. People may be living longer, but we've probably pushed longevity as far as it can go.
   AGREE   5   4   3   2   1   DISAGREE

2. I don't believe I should have to retire at 65; there's lots more I can accomplish.
   AGREE   5   4   3   2   1   DISAGREE

3. I rely on my doctor to keep me informed of the latest in medical and diet information.
   AGREE   5   4   3   2   1   DISAGREE

4. I already have set clear goals and objectives for 10
   years out.
   AGREE   5   4   3   2   1   DISAGREE

5. I check the nutritional content of all the food I eat.
   AGREE   5   4   3   2   1   DISAGREE

6. I consider myself an optimist.
   AGREE   5   4   3   2   1   DISAGREE

7. I have a good understanding of how exercise can benefit my health and life span.
   AGREE   5   4   3   2   1   DISAGREE

8. Despite all the hype about longevity, I think most
   people are still aging the way they always did.
   AGREE   5   4   3   2   1   DISAGREE

9. I like to pick unfamiliar destinations for my holiday
   travel.
   AGREE   5   4   3   2   1   DISAGREE

10. I don't see the point of having a bucket list. For me, at
    least, there probably won't be enough time.
    AGREE   5   4   3   2   1   DISAGREE

11. My faith matters to me.
    AGREE   5   4   3   2   1   DISAGREE

12. I'd like to start a business of my own someday.
    AGREE   5   4   3   2   1   DISAGREE

13. I am very worried about winding up in a nursing
    home.
    AGREE   5   4   3   2   1   DISAGREE

14. Even if you could live beyond 100, I don't think I'd want to.
    AGREE   5   4   3   2   1   DISAGREE

15. I am very interested in alternative and holistic medicine.
    AGREE   5   4   3   2   1   DISAGREE

16. I enjoy technology and try to keep up with the latest developments.
    AGREE   5   4   3   2   1   DISAGREE

17. I have already set clear goals and objectives for 20 years out.
    AGREE   5   4   3   2   1   DISAGREE

18. I've had a long and happy life, and it's time to relax and do nothing.
    AGREE   5   4   3   2   1   DISAGREE

19. I don't think there's much I can do to change my life.
    AGREE   5   4   3   2   1   DISAGREE

20. There are many new things I'd still like to learn.
    AGREE   5   4   3   2   1   DISAGREE

21. I don't see any reason I shouldn't expect to be at my grandchildren's weddings.
    AGREE   5   4   3   2   1   DISAGREE

22. There's a lot of buzz about "reversing aging," but I don't think it will ever really happen.
    AGREE   5   4   3   2   1   DISAGREE

23. I regularly seek out news about science and tech discoveries.
    AGREE   5   4   3   2   1   DISAGREE

24. I have already set clear goals and objectives for 30 years out.
    AGREE   5   4   3   2   1   DISAGREE

25. I am concerned about ageism and the tendency to discount what older generations can still contribute to society.
    AGREE   5   4   3   2   1   DISAGREE

As you can see, the quiz offers a mix of positive and negative statements; some describe a high state of awareness and concern, others, a low state; some describe an active and optimistic view of the future, others, more passive or even defeatist.

The benefit of the exercise is that it gets you to think about these topics all at once, and to reflect on their role in the aging process. These may be questions you haven't thought seriously about, or at all. What we're trying to do here, very simply, is to help you tune in to the idea of aging as a whole and begin to place it in the context of your own knowledge, attitudes, and beliefs.

There are no right or wrong answers and no need to add up or average your scores. The *thought process itself* is the whole point. What do you already know about these topics, how strongly do you feel about them, do they trigger any other thoughts or ideas about aging? Taking the quiz before you've read anything further will bring the DefaultAging versus SuperAging landscape into sharper focus and cause you to consider, and become more sensitive to, some of the key issues and options as they might affect you. That's all we're trying to accomplish at this stage.

GAIN A MICRO OUTLOOK

Here we look at the optimistic and pessimistic factors that *you* bring to the party based on your individual personality and independent of the topic of aging. We present the Life Orientation Test, originally developed at Carnegie Mellon University in 1985 and widely used for professional psychological assessments.

It's set up similar to our quiz on aging, with a series of statements and a five-point scale on which you can indicate the extent to which you agree or disagree. The scale places AGREE on the left and a continuum leading to DISAGREE on the right. Half the statements are expressed in the negative, so you would DISAGREE if you were an optimist; half the statements are expressed in the positive, so you would AGREE if you were an optimist. The reverse would be true if you were more of a pessimist. You can go through the quiz in just a few minutes. Read each statement and choose the number that matches your response. As with the first quiz, we recommend redoing it after you've read the book; for that reason, note your answers on a separate sheet of paper, and not directly in the text here.

1. I can find something meaningful or significant in everyday events.
   AGREE   5   4   3   2   1   DISAGREE

2. There is a reason for everything that happens to me.
   AGREE   5   4   3   2   1   DISAGREE

3. There is no ultimate meaning or purpose in life.
   AGREE   5   4   3   2   1   DISAGREE

4. There is no point in searching for meaning in life.
   AGREE   5   4   3   2   1   DISAGREE

5. No matter how painful the situation is, life is still worth living.
   AGREE   5   4   3   2   1   DISAGREE

6. The meaning of life is to "eat, drink, and be happy."
    AGREE   5   4   3   2   1   DISAGREE

7. What really matters to me is to pursue a higher pur-
    pose or calling, regardless of personal cost.
    AGREE   5   4   3   2   1   DISAGREE

8. I would rather be a happy pig than a sad saint.
    AGREE   5   4   3   2   1   DISAGREE

9. I am willing to sacrifice personal interests for the
    greater good.
    AGREE   5   4   3   2   1   DISAGREE

10. Personal happiness and success are more import-
    ant to me than achieving inner goodness and moral
    excellence.
    AGREE   5   4   3   2   1   DISAGREE

Your total score: _____
Your average (total / 10): _____

If your score averaged less than 3, you are more of a pessimist.

If you scored between 3 and 4, you're neutral and could go either way, depending on the situation.

If you scored 4 or more, you're inclined toward optimism and meaning in life.

Maybe you didn't need a test to tell you that you are more of a pessimist than an optimist. Or maybe you weren't sure, and you find your score to be revealing (and maybe disturbing). In either case, the question becomes: Can you change this?

Are you locked in to this set of attitudes? Is it possible to actually alter your personality?

An important pioneer in the field of positive psychology is Dr. Martin Seligman, an American psychologist, educator, and author. In 1967, Seligman began to study what he called "learned helplessness," when he discovered that in certain experiments, dogs did not respond to the opportunity to escape an unpleasant situation, even if they could. He theorized that people could *learn* to act helplessly, usually after failing to avoid a bad situation, even when they had the power to make things better. Seligman extended these findings to the study of clinical depression, arguing a major cause was an individual's perceived lack of control over an outcome.

This gradually led him to study the opposite: Can an individual learn to be positive? In 1990 he published *Learned Optimism*, which argued that a positive outlook can be consciously cultivated. This led to the positive psychology movement, of which Seligman is still a leader.

The key concept is response to adversity, codified as ABC: Adversity is an event that occurs; a Belief is then formed, interpreting that adverse event; and then there are Consequences, the actions and associated feelings that arise from the Belief.

Seligman's technique was to add a D and E component.

D stands for Disputation—consciously generating counter-evidence to the negative belief, in effect challenging it and talking yourself out of it. You might minimize the original adversity of the event or substitute a more positive belief by reminding yourself of the harmful effects of being negative. The point is, you don't let the negative belief stand unchallenged; you deliberately argue with it. E stands for Energization, which refers to the changes in both mood and outcome as a result of going through ABCD.

Seligman's method involves recording your mood and responses at each stage of the continuum. You describe a recent adversity (A), how you interpreted it (B), and what you felt and what you did as a result (C). You then write a counterargument (D) to the negative B, and then describe how it changed your energy (E).

Seligman's theories and methods are the foundation of the University of Pennsylvania's Master of Applied Positive Psychology program at the College of Liberal and Professional Studies. So, if you have to choose only one approach to train yourself to be more positive, we recommend the ABCDE method because of its underlying scientific credibility.

But let's not forget apps. There are literally hundreds of "positivity" apps available in both the Google and Apple stores. Many of them simply send you positive quotes every day. Some are digital versions of books, like Norman Vincent Peale's *The Power of Positive Thinking*. Others offer strategies and daily exercises. The field has become so vast that it's really a matter of checking it out for yourself and trying a few options.

Whether you try out ABCDE or discover a resource on your own, there are three key takeaways you should be aware of:

1. Attitude absolutely *can* extend your life. Being positive and having a specific purpose and goals are as important as physical health.
2. A positive Attitude toward SuperAging itself, with an active curiosity about its potential and a belief that it is indeed a revolution, will set you up to be able to realize all the pillars more effectively.
3. If your natural inclination is toward pessimism, you *can* change this. If you're already an optimist, you can and should reinforce this and make it even stronger. Either way, you should practice a positive-thinking booster program *every single day*.

FAKE IT AND YOU'LL MAKE IT?

One final tip, and we find it to be a very intriguing idea. You may be able to create a more positive Attitude simply by acting as if your Attitude was more positive.

This theory was developed most famously by Amy Cuddy, an American psychologist, author, and speaker who developed the concept of "power posing." She based her technique on the premise that how you hold your body strongly influences how you feel and behave. An open or expansive stance, making you appear taller and wider, makes you feel more powerful; a posture of contraction, more hunched or defensive, makes you feel less powerful. Her bottom line: stand up straight, smile, look like you're in charge. Adopting and holding a power pose for as little as two minutes can work wonders, she argues.

Cuddy's presentation of this concept at a TED conference went on to become the second most-viewed TED talk of all time, and her book on the topic became a bestseller translated into more than 30 languages. We should note that her theory is not without controversy, particularly as she claimed that the posing technique actually triggers hormonal changes that can be measured. According to her critics, blind studies have failed to replicate this evidence. But even without clinical proof of beneficial physical change, the follow-up research did appear to validate the end result.

Try it and see for yourself!

3

AWARENESS

Attitude is the first foundational element of the SuperAging tool kit, offering an exciting vision of future possibilities and creating the energy to go after it. Without this Attitude, the full potential of SuperAging can never be realized.

But Awareness is just as important.

There has always been a flow of information, to some extent, about aging. Up until very recently, however, it has overwhelmingly been focused on one thing: living longer—i.e., physical health. DefaultAgers have certainly been interested in the topic, and books on diet and exercise have been around for a long time, and have morphed (along with every other topic of communication) into websites, blogs, YouTube videos, and social media posts. If the focus is strictly limited to how to add more years, there isn't much difference between what DefaultAgers and SuperAgers might know (or be able to learn).

But is "adding more years" the beginning and end of the topic? After all, our SuperAging mantra is "Getting older without getting old." The "getting older" part presupposes living longer.

It's the second part—"without getting old"—that creates a whole new level of requirement when it comes to Awareness. Now there are many more topics to keep track of, above and beyond physical health or numerical longevity.

To fully maximize the promise of SuperAging, you need to start paying attention to how you are going to spend those extra years so that you are not "old." And that in turn means dealing with everything from retirement and personal reinvention to housing, to financial strategies, to relationships, to technology . . . and more.

So when we say Awareness, we're simply talking about this expanded list of subjects. Let's compare how this list might look for DefaultAgers and SuperAgers.

	DEFAULTAGERS	SUPERAGERS
Underlying premise	"If I'm 65, I probably haven't got that many years left, but at least let them be as free from pain and hardship as possible."	"If I'm 65, I could easily be looking at another 20 or 30 years, and I want them to be as fulfilling as possible."
Resulting focus for Awareness	PHYSICAL HEALTH A few more years (if possible) Less pain and hardship	PHYSICAL HEALTH *Many* more years (if I keep up to date with and pursue all that's possible) BUT ALSO What I need to know to make those years dynamic, productive, exciting—i.e., "Getting older without getting old"
Topics to be aware of	PHYSICAL HEALTH Medications Diet Fitness GOVERNMENT BENEFITS	PHYSICAL HEALTH Medications Diet Fitness Prevention New research Technology aids HOUSING Aging in place Relocation? Technology RETIREMENT Keep working? New career? Education Reinvention RELATIONSHIPS Existing network New networks? FINANCIAL STRATEGIES Need a whole new approach if I think I will live to 100

DEFAULTAGER VERSUS SUPERAGER LEARNING

DefaultAgers are essentially passive about information. The approach is mostly to let the information come to them as opposed to actively seeking it out. This is particularly true of medical information that relates to their own condition. For most DefaultAgers, this information is in the hands of their doctor—and their doctor, whose authority is supreme and unchallenged, will tell them what they need to know.

This even applies to their own personal data. Most don't know, at any given time, their own blood pressure, cholesterol level, blood sugar level, other readings derived from blood tests, or other vital health measurements. It's up to the doctor to keep the appropriate records and alert them if there are any concerns. The idea that they would want to possess all this data themselves, much less manage it by tracking or updating on a regular basis, is, at best, very weakly held.

Consequently, they have a very narrow range of resources that can contribute information about aging in general, and their own condition in particular (especially when it comes to future prospects or opportunities that they may not have considered). They may be on the internet, but they do not follow any systematic program of information-gathering and evaluation. It's not that they are indifferent to the information, it's that their level of Awareness is determined by whatever happens to make its way in.

SuperAgers, by contrast, approach Awareness from a proactive point of view and are much more likely to actively seek it.

This sets up three big contrasts with the DefaultAgers.

1. Reluctance to see "experts" as the sole source. The doctor (particularly, the first-line GP or family doctor) is respected, but is not seen as an unimpeachable source, let alone the sole source. SuperAgers want more points of view—from other physicians, from medical websites, even from fellow sufferers of the same medical conditions. For example, the website PatientsLikeMe tracks over 2,800 conditions and enables users to meet and engage with others in the same situation. There are numerous similar websites specializing in just one condition, like diabetes or heart and stroke issues.

2. Determination to know and control their own personal health data. As noted above, DefaultAgers accept that the doctor is the gatekeeper of their medical data. They're not interested in keeping their own test results, X-rays, and other key information. Isn't all that up to their physician? Besides, how would they get hold of all that data, and what would they do once they had it? But SuperAgers don't accept those limitations. To them, Awareness extends to their own health information (in fact, it might even begin there). They are much more ready and willing to explore personalized electronic health records, for which there are now a huge number of products and systems available, and to use apps (hundreds now available) to monitor and track their own key health metrics. For the SuperAger, Awareness definitely extends to intimately knowing what is happening in your own body.

3. Readiness to use multiple resources to get the information they need. SuperAgers don't want to wait for the necessary information to come to them; they're ready and willing to seek it out through every means available, particularly the internet. They have a higher rate of internet usage (including social media) than DefaultAgers, and they are more familiar with search techniques and the use of forums or other means of dialogue that may deliver information from nontraditional (i.e., *not* mass media) sources.

The two groups, then, have dramatically different understandings of what the word "Awareness" encompasses when it comes to aging, and what's required to achieve and maintain a satisfactory level of Awareness.

It doesn't follow, of course, that all SuperAgers necessarily have the skills to do what they'd like to do. Or that their desire to be more proactive when it comes to Awareness necessarily translates into an organized system they can practice consistently.

That's where this book comes in.

It's not enough for you to want to know more, or even to be ready and willing to go and get more. As never before, Awareness requires a set of skills and a structure for applying them. That's what makes Awareness a **working tool** and not just a vaguely desirable goal.

If we start out by confronting the total information landscape—before we do any selecting, categorizing, or any other organizing—it can look like a completely chaotic and intimidating jungle of topics. On any given day, you may find yourself googling questions like these:

- What's the latest technology to help me age at home?
- What are the best side hustles for people over the age of 50?
- What is the latest research on how to prevent dementia?
- What's the latest research on organ regeneration and replacement?
- How are they using AI to promote longevity?
- What are the 10 best places to retire to?
- Am I at serious risk of outliving my money?
- Why are so many Baby Boomers getting divorced?
- Do I need a "lifestyle reinvention" coach, and if so, who are the best ones?
- What universities offer programs for retirees?
- Why do scientists think they will be able to reverse aging?

And this is, of course, only a minute sample of what the information torrent looks like. Some of the topics come as no surprise. Health and fitness are good examples: we expect that a lot of information would be out there, we know it's relevant to the topic of aging, and we can readily go looking for it.

But there are many other topics we may be only vaguely aware of, or not at all. We may spot an occasional article on some astonishing new lab research to slow down or reverse aging, but we may not realize that so much is going on in that field that it's worth our while to treat it as a category of constant attention. The same goes for robotics or AI. We may not even be thinking about these. Or about aging in place, or second acts and career reinvention, or the latest ideas in how to solve the problem of outliving your money.

Yet these topics are essential to having a full picture of what SuperAging could be, and how to achieve it. We need to make sure we're keeping an eye on them—and the best way to do that is to have an organized tracking system.

MAKE AWARENESS PART OF YOUR SUPERAGING PROGRAM

The system we recommend has four components:

- Create a list of SuperAging topics
- Choose your sources
- Select and store your content
- Vet your sources

CREATE A LIST OF SUPERAGING TOPICS

The first step is to list the major SuperAging topics you'll be following. Of course, there are literally thousands of possibilities, but we recommend keeping it simple and using large and intuitive categories. All of these play into at least one of the seven *A*'s; some touch on several.

1. **Diet:** Healthy eating, foods that promote longevity, recipes, and menu plans
2. **Fitness:** Physical and mental health, including exercise programs and brain fitness programs
3. **Finance:** Investment strategies, financial independence
4. **Health:** Prevention and wellness, anti-aging research, new therapies, new products and services for monitoring and tracking
5. **Housing:** Aging in place and associated products and services, healthy locations for retirement, new concepts in retirement living and senior housing
6. **People:** Human-interest stories about SuperAgers, role models
7. **Relationships:** Social connectivity, new technology (e.g., AI, robots), apps, and other digital tools
8. **Retirement:** Retirement planning, new forms of retirement (part-time, hybrid, second careers, and reinvention), new forms of ongoing activity (volunteering, mentoring), techniques for long-term planning
9. **Science:** Biomedical research, new projects, and discoveries related to slowing down, preventing, or reversing aging

10. **Social issues:** Politics, combating ageism, economic
    and demographic trends that influence the other
    topics
11. **Technology:** Age-tech (including telehealth and
    interactive monitoring), AI, robotics, cloud-based
    interconnected systems

Your own list may vary. Feel free to add more or to relabel or
redefine some of the categories to make them more descriptive
or applicable to your particular priorities. You may also add or
subtract, or regroup; as time goes on, it's inevitable that new
topics will emerge.

CHOOSE YOUR SOURCES

Our list of topics gives us a consistent structure to organize the
information landscape, but we also need a way to categorize all
the sources from which information can flow. We quickly see
that there are two types of sources:

- **Core sources that focus specifically on aging and
  related issues.** These may be books, publications,
  websites, YouTube channels, blogs, podcasts,
  e-newsletters, etc. Some may have the dissemination
  of information as their main purpose; others may
  be the websites or publication arms of aging-related
  organizations (e.g., AARP or, in Canada, CARP) that
  have wider agendas than information only. Together,
  they represent a "core" list of sources that we will
  want to check on a regular basis.
- **Intermittent sources that do not focus on aging,
  but which may offer valuable information from**

time to time. The topic of aging is becoming so important that virtually all media—from the *New York Times* to *Newsweek* to the *Economist* to *Forbes*—regularly produce articles, blog posts, or videos with new and important information on one of our key topics. How do you find this information if you're not regularly following those publications?

CORE SOURCES

For the core group, we can develop a simple table that lists the sources we are checking regularly:

TOPICS	DESCRIPTION	"CORE GROUP" SOURCES					
		BOOKS	NEWSPAPERS, MAGAZINES	WEBSITES, E-NEWS-LETTERS	VIDEO, PODCASTS	APPS	OTHER
SUPERAGING	The whole topic overall						
DIET	Healthier eating, cooking, menu plans						
FITNESS	Exercise programs, best practices						
FINANCE	Investment, financial independence						
HEALTH	Prevention, treatment, overall wellness						
HOUSING	Aging in place						
PEOPLE	Human-interest stories, role models						

Of course, there could be many more topics than just the six we have laid out here. Each would get its own line in the chart.

Possibilities include: Relationships, Retirement, Science, Social Issues, Technology. Your list will probably expand over time as you learn more and new subjects come into view. Here's what it might start to look like with a few specific entries:

TOPICS	DESCRIPTION	"CORE GROUP" SOURCES					
		BOOKS	NEWSPAPERS, MAGAZINES	WEBSITES, E-NEWS-LETTERS	VIDEO, PODCASTS	APPS	OTHER
SUPERAGING	The whole topic overall	*Ageless: The New Science of Getting Older Without Getting Old*		SuperAging.info, AARP.com, Theaging-academy.com	*Live Long and Master Aging, Knowledge-able Aging, Living to 100 Club*		
DIET	Healthier eating, cooking, menu plans			BlueZones.com		SeniorFit-ness, OverFifty Fitness	
FITNESS	Exercise programs, best practices	*Workouts for Seniors Over 60*		BabyBoom-ers.com			
FINANCE	Investment, financial indepen-dence	*The 100-Year Life*					
HEALTH	Prevention, treatment, overall wellness	*Younger You*		WebMD, MedicalX-press		LifeExtend, Qardio Health	
HOUSING	Aging in place			SeniorHous-ingNews.com, Ageinplace-tech.com			
PEOPLE	Human-interest stories, role models						

At this point, you may be wondering how complicated this needs to be. Are you expected to fill in every blank all at once? Should you be checking the list weekly? Monthly? Is there software that can help?

A good analogy is to look at financial management software. There are thousands of people who use Quicken, for example, to track literally every transaction, no matter how small or routine.

Many others rebel at this kind of micro-tracking, arguing that it can too easily become obsessive and impossible to maintain. Should they really be worrying about a coffee at Starbucks that they neglected to enter into the system? They limit their use of the financial management software to major issues like overall budgeting and cash flow or taxes, and they don't sweat the small stuff.

The latter, simpler approach is better, at least to start with.

It's important to remember that we're talking about Awareness here, not encyclopedic knowledge. The simple act of *looking* at the chart periodically—even once every three or four weeks—provides an immediate reminder of the topics themselves. Gradually you'll become more and more familiar with the list, and more and more aware of your own frequency of checking up on your sources. You'll develop a feel for how long it's been since you saw something or read something on a given topic, and whether you're generally up to date with the latest wisdom.

Your own interests and predispositions are important too. You'll soon find it's impossible to be equally aware of every topic, and that your level of attention will vary widely. There's nothing wrong with this! Remember, what you're comparing this to is a previous condition in which you had no list of topics, no list of sources, no systematic way of going after the information you need. By keeping it simple, you're more likely to get into the habit of checking up on a regular basis instead of being burdened by a task list that never quite gets satisfied. Being a SuperAger does require work, but it shouldn't be overly complex or burdensome. Keep it simple to begin with and find your own comfort level for how frequently you track and update.

INTERMITTENT SOURCES

Your core group of regularly scanned sources, robust as it may be, represents only a fraction of the information that's out there on any given topic. There will be a virtual fire hose of articles, blogs, videos, podcasts, and so on coming from sources that are not listed in your core resources library. To get a handle on this flood, we recommend digital alerts.

Alert systems are operated by third-party services that search the web and alert you when a topic appears that matches a search term you specify. There are many services that offer this. Our two favorites (Google Alerts and Talkwalker Alerts) are free; others charge monthly fees but offer more robust features, including the ability to analyze what you're receiving.

But at the simplest level, which is what we'll stick to here, you basically compile a list of search terms you're interested in. Whenever something appears on the internet that matches one of your search terms, the service sends you an email alert and a link to where the term appears (article, video, podcast, etc.). You can specify how often you want to receive alerts. You can also let them accumulate in your email inbox and check them when convenient. The important thing is that the services are constantly examining the internet for material that contains your search terms.

David uses Google Alerts, and here is the list of search terms he's currently using:

- BABY BOOMERS
- LIVING TO 100
- RETIREMENT
- WORKING PAST RETIREMENT
- AGE-TECH
- REVERSE AGING

- LONGEVITY
- REINVENTING AGING
- CENTENARIANS
- OUTLIVING YOUR MONEY
- HEALTH TECH
- AGEISM

The list may not look that big, and that's by design. You should keep the list small, especially at the beginning: you don't want to get overwhelmed and see hundreds of results piling up in your email inbox and be unable to deal with them. As you go along, you can drop certain search terms or add others, such as subtopics of subjects producing results that you find particularly interesting or helpful.

SELECT AND STORE YOUR CONTENT

Okay, we now have content pouring in, but we need one more vitally important tool: some method of selecting the content we want to keep and putting it somewhere where we can review it at our convenience. Does this mean you shouldn't read the inbound material right away? Not at all! Depending on what it is and how it engages you (and what else you have going on at the time), you may indeed want to jump on a given article or new video immediately.

But in practice, you're going to receive more than you can handle on an as-you-go-along basis. You need to find some way to select what's most useful so you can review it in more detail at your convenience. Ideally, you should be able to annotate it or move it to a specific topic-defined folder rather than having it all sit there as a mass. Once in your storage system, the content can be saved as a permanent reference or culled and deleted when appropriate. You should be able to move this content in and out of storage constantly, as needed. Finally, you should be able to access it from multiple devices (laptop, tablet, phone).

Fortunately, there are good existing systems that will enable you to do all this. We recommend three for your consideration: Evernote, Nimbus Note, and Notion. All three create a digital workspace where your selected content can be stored. Very importantly, since so much of that content will be in the form of a web page (be it an article, blog, podcast, or video), all three offer a browser plug-in that works as a "web clipper," enabling you to immediately save that web page directly into the workspace. No need to manually copy the material and paste it into a document or file.

Once it's in the workspace, more can be done with an item than to just have it on a list. You can convert a single large, undifferentiated list into any number of sub-lists, by topic or date or any other criterion. You can link related items. You can create additional, independent functions such as task lists, calendars, and project management systems. Visit SuperAging.info and check the Resources section for more information on how and where to get specific online training for these features, and for other systems that can enable you to do the same thing. For now, though, let's just leave it as a very simple way to capture your reading as you go along, and to store it for convenient review later.

To sum up: We've gone from a crowded and confused landscape where the information is pouring in on us from every direction, disorganized and undifferentiated, to a workspace or notebook where we've captured and categorized only what really matters. We started with a topics framework to identify the big categories we're watching, then used an alerts system to snag all the information that fits search terms we ourselves have created, and added a web clipper feature to quickly move entire relevant web pages into a digital storage vault for periodic review.

One big question remains: How do we know which information can be trusted?

VET YOUR SOURCES

No matter how we organize the inbound torrent or how cleverly we categorize and select and then store our selections in an orderly vault for later review and evaluation, the fact remains that some of it will be more reliable and some will be less reliable. That's just a fact of life in the internet age.

The topic of misinformation is particularly hot right now, given the political climate and the frequent suspension of social media and YouTube accounts (whether justified or not) on the grounds that they are trafficking in misinformation.

Our advice is: Relax. It can be handled. We recommend a very short and simple list of vetting practices:

Use social media *only* as a jumping-off point. Social media should never be a source by itself. Social media can refer you to a source, which can then be viewed and evaluated.

Look at who is giving an endorsement. If you're reading a book, check out the qualifications of those who are recommending it. If reviewers or endorsers have relevant credentials, it's more likely the content is reliable. Don't forget that "relevant credentials" may include being a fellow SuperAger; some books may be factually accurate but too technical, so if some of the endorsements come from readers who have enjoyed the work and found it useful, this can and should be a factor in your own evaluation.

Be wary of definitive conclusions around emerging data. Be cautious of conclusions that are too definitive too early on, particularly when it comes to constantly updating science and research. (COVID is a particularly nasty and instructive example of what happens when incomplete or fast-changing information is presented as final and conclusive fact.)

Trust reputable, proven sources. Prefer sources that are backed by solid and documented research from blue-chip institutions. Be suspicious of "gurus" with oversimplified advice based solely on their own anecdotal experience.

Make room for differing opinions. Don't be afraid of uncertainty, gray areas, or even contradictory evidence or conclusions. What you should be trying to do is weed out what is clearly bogus. There's plenty of room for differing opinions or emerging research that adds new light to subjects. To take one example: a very hot topic right now is the possibility of reversing aging by turning off senescent cells. But how far away is a real application? Some scientists say 10 years; some say 20 or 30. (Only a very few, interestingly enough, say never.) Diverging views such as these may be equally reliable expressions of reasonable differences in current knowledge and judgment. You don't want to stifle the excitement and creativity of exploring this wonderful landscape; the fact that it is fast-changing is part of what makes it so important and valuable. SuperAging is the most profound social revolution we have ever seen, so it's not surprising that it's an arena for vigorous debate.

Make a habit of checking in with SuperAging.info. We mentioned our companion website before, but it bears repeating. We've worked hard to patrol and analyze the jungle of information and curate the material that is most trustworthy and reliable. It's an ongoing effort, of course, because so much new material is coming out all the time. To keep your Awareness skills acute and current, this book and our website are your partners.

These vetting practices are good to keep in mind as you deal with all the inbound content. But there is one final element that is the most important of all: Attitude and Awareness are the foundational necessities, the two bedrock *A*'s of SuperAging because they equip us to engage with the other pillars, all of which are more specific in their roles and applications. It's now time to examine each of them in detail.

4

ACTIVITY

The first two *A*'s—Attitude and Awareness—are foundational to the whole SuperAging idea because they spill over to affect all the other components. Armed with a SuperAger's Attitude toward the aging process itself and equipped with the tools to create and maintain a high level of Awareness in a crowded information landscape, you can now engage with the other *A*'s, each of which has a more specific focus.

First comes Activity.

Technically, everything you do could be called Activity, whether it deals with your body or your finances or your social network or your career. But in the context of SuperAging, we define Activity as meaning physical or mental activity to promote health and well-being. This covers:

- Wellness (which encompasses overall health and disease prevention or mitigation)
- Diet and nutrition
- Exercise and physical fitness

- Brain health, especially prevention or mitigation of dementia/Alzheimer's disease

All these topics are already rich with information—books, websites, YouTube channels, apps. In fact, there is almost too much information on health and well-being, and not surprisingly, some of it includes sharp differences of opinion about which approaches are "best." More carbs or more proteins? What about peptides? What about supplements? What about fasting? Walking or weight training, or both? Do brain games really work, or are you just fooling yourself?

In choosing how best to navigate this forest of fact and judgment, we are guided by a few basic principles. Everything we present:

- Is endorsed by credible experts and, where possible, backed up by scientific research.
- Can achieve positive results. Are there are other things that can also produce good results? Of course. If we covered all that's out there, we could produce a 5,000-page chapter on diet alone! We had to be selective, but we continue to search and analyze and update (another important reason to follow SuperAging.info).
- Is workable. You *can* do this!
- Can be done at home. We deliberately excluded expensive equipment or the need to visit expensive facilities. Of course, if you already have a home gym or are working out at a fitness club or have a personal trainer, you should absolutely continue! But you *can* be a SuperAger without following complex systems or incurring high costs.
- Is intended to serve as a road map, an aid, and

hopefully, an inspiration toward learning more and keeping your knowledge up to date. But it's not a rigid system or set of rules requiring you to do every single thing. Most importantly, it is *not* intended to replace medical advice, so be sure to check with your doctor before following any particular diet or exercise program.

TOTAL LIFESTYLE APPROACHES

Wellness, diet and nutrition, exercise and physical fitness, and brain health are typically treated as four distinct topics, each with its own set of experts and information. But there is also a way of integrating them seamlessly into an overall lifestyle.

THE BLUE ZONES

The Blue Zones Project was developed by author, journalist, and explorer Dan Buettner, who led a *National Geographic* team of medical researchers, demographers, and anthropologists to discover the secrets of longevity by analyzing areas that already had a disproportionate number of people living to 100. (The benchmark was that people had to reach the age of 100 at a rate that was 10 times greater than the United States as a whole.)

Were there such communities? And if so, were there any common denominators in the attitudes and behaviors of their populations? This was the key to the whole project, because Buettner's team knew from research like the Danish twin study (1996) that genes probably determine only about 20% of how long a person lives. The rest is environment and lifestyle. If the team could identify long-living communities, and if they then could discover attitudes and behaviors that were common to those communities, this could serve as a model that could be universally applied.

The team succeeded on both levels. First they identified five communities:

1. The Barbagia region of Sardinia, which has the world's highest concentration of male centenarians.
2. Ikaria, Greece, an island with one of the world's lowest rates of middle-age mortality.
3. Nicoya Peninsula, Costa Rica, another area with one of the world's lowest rates of middle-age mortality, as well as the world's second-highest concentration of male centenarians.
4. Loma Linda, California, specifically, the Seventh-day Adventist community, members of which live 10 years longer than the North American average.
5. Okinawa, Japan, where the female population over 70 is the longest-lived group in the world.

They then identified nine common-denominator attitudes and behaviors, which Buettner dubbed Power 9. This led not only to the publication of a bestseller but to a mini-industry, with follow-up books, a website, education programs, and an active public policy program working with other communities to create environments that could promote longevity along the lines of Power 9.

Here are the Power 9 components:

1. **Move naturally.** The people in Blue Zone communities live in environments that "constantly nudge them into moving without thinking about it." For example, they don't use modern technology to aid in house and yard work.

2. **Have a purpose.** On Okinawa, it's *ikigai*; for the Nicoyans, it's *plan de vida*. According to the Blue Zone researchers, having a sense of purpose can be worth seven extra years of life expectancy.

3. **Downshift.** Blue Zone people try to reduce stress, whether that means taking a little time each day to think about their ancestors, praying, napping, or observing happy hour.

4. **Follow the 80% rule for eating.** Okinawans stop eating when their stomachs are 80% full. In all the Blue Zone communities as a whole, people eat their smallest meal in late afternoon or early evening and then don't eat for the rest of the day.

5. **Follow a largely plant-based diet.** Beans are the most important component of the Blue Zoners' diets. Meat is eaten only about five times per month.

6. **Drink a moderate amount of alcohol.** Blue Zoners (except Adventists, who abstain altogether) drink one to two glasses per day (mostly wine).

7. **Be part of a faith-based community.** In the Attitude chapter, we noted that there seems to be a statistical correlation between faith and longevity. This certainly applies to the Blue Zone communities. Over 90% of Blue Zone centenarians belong to a faith-based community; there is no significance to denomination.

8. **Focus on families.** Blue Zone centenarians put their families first, keeping aging parents or grandparents close by (or right in the home). Most have committed to a life partner and are heavily invested in their children.

9. **Maintain strong social networks.** Blue Zone centenarians belong to social circles that reinforce healthy

behaviors. Okinawans actually create groups of five friends who commit to each other for life.

You can see that five of the Power 9 items do not relate to diet or exercise but involve other important behaviors that are part of the Attachment component of our seven *A*'s program. We'll go into this in a lot more detail in that chapter.

But in focusing on the exercise piece, what's striking is that the beneficial behaviors flow naturally from the overall lifestyle itself. They are not external actions jarringly brought into a daily routine. You don't stop your regular life to briefly do a workout; your physical activity is an ongoing part of that regular life.

This does *not* mean that workouts are bad! When you exercise, you do interrupt your regular life by changing your clothes, location, and bodily activity. In fact, that deliberate change is part of the whole idea; you certainly can't lift those weights or ride that bike for more than a (relatively) brief and concentrated period of time. But what the Blue Zone example does show is that we can—and emphatically should—incorporate physical activity into our regular life much more consistently and even unobtrusively, so that the workouts, if we do them, are not the only physical activity we are getting. More on this below.

As to diet, the Blue Zone example does represent a very definite program of what's in and what's out, and not all of us may be able to (or want to) follow it. But the underlying principles—less filling meals in the evening, less meat, alcohol in moderation—are becoming much more widely accepted.

The Blue Zone philosophy is being applied across a wide range of subtopics, even including home design. The idea is that your entire environment is at once your arena, your supporter, and your coach. Longevity-boosting attitudes and behaviors occur not as external elements brought into an otherwise neutral (or even hostile) environment, but as inherent features of that environment. (We'll have more to say about the Blue Zone influence on home design in the chapter on Autonomy.)

BIOHACKING

Blue Zone isn't the only total lifestyle approach that is making news. Another growing phenomenon is biohacking. Though somewhat controversial because it can involve drastic interventions in your physical and mental health, it's an instructive manifestation of the SuperAging drive to exert more influence and control over outcomes without always relying on conventional medicine. We think you should at least know about it, if only to increase your understanding of what's going on out there. But at the same time, be careful.

Essentially, biohacking covers a wide range of manipulations in body and brain, ranging from dietary modifications to attempts to modify DNA to bodily implants. There are three categories of biohacking:

1. **Nutrigenomics.** Nutrigenomics goes beyond general "good" dietary principles and focuses on the inter-action between your genes and the foods you eat. It tests how different nutrients affect your health, and usually results in a dietary regimen including many supplements, with the goal of improving your body's gene expression. Advocates claim it can reduce the risk of developing certain diseases, promote weight loss, and produce healthier gut bacteria.
2. **DIYbio.** Here we up the ante and try to modify DNA. This usually requires the participation of trained medical professionals, although some of the necessary equipment is now more widely available.

Processes include extracting your own DNA, testing it, and preparing bacteria cultures to create genetically modified organisms. Not surprisingly, it's very controversial because of the risk of unqualified people carrying out these activities.

3. **Grinders.** Grinding involves actual body modifications, carried out by professionals. These include injections and implants, including the implanting of computer chips in the body. There is a significant amount of expert opinion that the real key to longevity will be the blurring of the line between human and machine, or transhumanism. Yes, it's a real idea, and it has attracted billions in investment!

As you can see, biohacking covers a wide range, from slightly more intensive dietary practices all the way to the fringes of making us bionic humans. It certainly captures the spirit of SuperAging, feeding into the idea that we can and should take more control over health and longevity. Traditional medicine, on the other hand, is slower, more gradual, and largely reactive ("sick care" rather than healthcare). So biohacking is psychologically very attractive.

The question is: Is it safe? (Is it even legal?)

The answer can be complicated. At the safe and legal end of the spectrum, biohacking has led to many beneficial products and practices like better diet and exercise programs, deeper appreciation of the importance of sleep, the benefits of meditation, and even the development of wearable technology. And where supplements are concerned, there is already considerable regulation, and some, like steroids, are banned. As for the more extreme solutions, in the United States, the Food and Drug Administration is starting to take a closer look at genetic engineering and who is doing it. Right now the focus is on preventing access to gene testing and editing "kits" for untrained people, but we expect to see increased regulatory attention and activity in the future.

One of the underlying biohacking ideas that is likely to grow is the concept of increased personalization, that your DNA may produce different health risks and responses to diet or drugs than the DNA of someone else. The ultimate goal is a highly individualized program tailored to your unique bodily makeup. This is the subject of a great deal of research, and we can expect many more positive developments not limited to prevention (which is essentially what biohacking is all about) but also extending to treatments and therapies. The trick is to be aware of them, to keep up to date with the new thinking but at the same time realize that *not all of these approaches may work as advertised*, and that new research will continue to produce new insights and better methods.

Bottom line: Employ Awareness of this topic by adding it to your search topics so you can keep your eye on its evolution and *be realistic and objective* about its potential. The Resources section at SuperAging.info includes some essential reading and websites to check out.

As we've seen, then, whether it's a relatively gentler approach like Blue Zones or a more intense one like biohacking, there is widespread interest in the total lifestyle concept rather than a single-issue focus like a new miracle diet or exercise plan.

That said, we can also proceed on a topic-by-topic basis to find new thinking and valuable ideas. Let's now look at each of the four components of Activity—wellness, diet and nutrition, exercise and physical fitness, and brain health—with a goal of curating some essentials and finding what's new or what may be a new spin on an old topic that you haven't thought about.

WELLNESS

When it comes to your healthcare, can you behave like a *consumer*?

In the DefaultAging world, the question would have been impossible. You're a *patient*, not a consumer. The professional medical community—doctors, nurses, hospitals, insurance companies—controls the landscape. Yes, there are protections such as privacy laws and malpractice regulations, but your range of options is very limited. You don't even have access to your own data.

As for competition, forget it. Although there is a constant swarm of innovative activity on the research side, the delivery side is sclerotic. There is no culture of customer service. You have to accept whatever the system chooses to deliver, and pay whatever the system charges.

But not anymore.

The biggest revolution of the SuperAging world—far bigger than any miracle diet or magic workout plan—is the **consumerization of healthcare**. SuperAgers are starting to behave toward the healthcare system the same way they behave (and have always behaved) toward other consumer-driven industries: they shop around, demand options, voice complaints, and support new ideas and better service.

In other words, SuperAgers are taking more control of their own health and healthcare.

The new reality was well summed up in a report by *Insider Intelligence*: "The consumerization of healthcare . . . is threatening hospitals' bottom lines." The report noted that rather than being passive recipients of healthcare, patients had shifted into becoming active participants, reviewing doctors online, visiting their local CVS instead of going to the hospital or urgent care, and not being afraid to switch providers based on their experiences.

The signs are everywhere.

Primary care 24/7. Innovative new services are challenging the accepted models. For example, the service 98point6 enables 24/7 text-based consultation with primary care physicians at no cost or low cost. The same kind of approach can be found at One Medical, which delivers primary care at 125 locations and offers 24/7 virtual service. That care includes same day or next day long-slot appointments (in person or virtual) and drop-in lab services. Appointments that start on time? And that last longer so you don't feel rushed? Welcome to the new reality.

Consumer reporting. There is a proliferation of websites that report on healthcare from a consumer, not a clinician, point of view. At sites like RateMDs or Healthgrades, you can rate your own doctor, or check the ratings of doctors you are considering. Both sites claim ratings on close to three million doctors. You can also consult directly with other patients. There are websites with interactive chat rooms specializing in virtually every disease or large all-in-one place sites such as PatientsLikeMe that claim 850,000 members tracking over 2,800 different medical conditions.

P4P (pay for performance). Also known as value-based payment, P4P creates models that attach both incentives and disincentives to provider performance, tying reimbursement to measurable results. P4P started with hospital reimbursement, with rewards for excellent performance (not just clinical outcomes, but also a variety of patient-satisfaction metrics) and penalties for subpar performance (including unacceptably high rates of readmission). It's now widespread as a model to reimburse individual doctors as well. As far back as 2017, for example, the largest health insurers in the United States,

Aetna and UnitedHealth Group, reported that nearly half their reimbursements were via some form of value-based models.

The medical profession has responded too, particularly in the area of family practice, which is the most patient-facing sector. More practices are offering concierge-type services designed to improve patient satisfaction by morphing from transaction-based (one appointment followed by the next appointment) to more holistic relationships, including after-hours service, integration of in-office and telehealth visits, and more assistance to the patient in navigating the entire healthcare system.

Larger institutions are also responding. Many hospitals, for example, have patient websites where patients can view their charts, medications, and appointments. There seems to be a recognition that the patient can be and *should be* an active and knowledgeable participant in the healthcare process.

Electronic health record systems. These are enabling more people to gain access to their own medical data, while numerous apps and wearables empower people to monitor and track key metrics like pulse, blood pressure, and blood sugar. These systems also make it easier for both physicians and hospitals to deliver vital records and relevant information to patients.

Upscale healthcare. Just as retailing includes both mass marketers and upscale luxury stores, the same segmentation is happening in healthcare, and SuperAgers are getting particular attention. One good example is Human Longevity, which offers a membership program called 100+, specifically designed to help people reach the century mark. President David Karow was quoted in an article in *Worth*: "Our battle cry is 'Die young as late as you can!'" Members receive a personal physician, testing to predict risk of disease, and access to specialists. Originally based in San Diego, Human Longevity has plans to expand around the world. Too expensive? Dr. Karow explained his company's goal of democratizing precision medicine and belief that options that may be impractical for many patients now will one day be affordable and conventional. His company's clients, he says, are the pioneers.

These developments haven't happened abruptly; they've been coming for a long time. One of the earliest to forecast this change was Sir Muir Gray, whose long and distinguished career in the United Kingdom included being the chief knowledge officer for the National Health Service and earning a knighthood for creating the National Library for Health. In 2001, he coauthored *The Resourceful Patient*, which explained why the power of clinicians was going to decline and the power of patients, morphing into consumers, was going to increase. He updated the book in 2015, to reflect the astonishing pace of change propelled in part by the internet.

Sir Muir envisions a whole new paradigm for healthcare in the 21st century, "a transformation of the way in which medicine is practiced and healthcare delivered." The transformation would be characterized by shared decision-making between patient and clinician, and patients would be equipped with resources "that would allow them to manage their care to a much greater degree than is possible at present." He imagines "a resourceful patient" preparing in advance for a consultation with the doctor "by reading material available on the web and by ensuring that all the terms, concerns, and options that may come up during the consultation are understood."

All these changes, both in attitude and behavior, are driven by the SuperAgers' concern with *wellness* as the important overriding goal, as opposed to the DefaultAging model where *treatment* is the dominant force. In the DefaultAging world, you get sick, you get treated, you're better—one, two, three—and then don't encounter the healthcare system until the next time you get sick. Healthcare is just individual transactions delivered by (real or perceived) totally qualified experts to totally unqualified recipients.

But once the lens changes to wellness, everything else follows. Wellness implies consistent and comprehensive attention, even absent a specific illness or complaint. And who better to pay that attention than you? You become the captain, the driver of your own overall health.

True, you call on the professionals to treat episodes of illness. But importantly, you're still engaged the rest of the time. You're interested in prevention, more consistent monitoring, discovering newer and better methods of . . . well, everything. Including how and where treatment is delivered and whether there are better options. As a SuperAger, you're an active manager, not a passive recipient.

MAKE WELLNESS PART OF YOUR SUPERAGING PROGRAM

RECOGNIZE THAT THE WORLD HAS CHANGED

This is simply a matter of realizing there's more potential for you to take charge than you may have thought. You still need to be careful and methodical, of course, but at least make sure you're armed with this new mindset. You have a lot more room to take action, and there are a lot more resources to help you.

REALIZE YOU HAVE CHOICES

Think about your own healthcare experiences and reimagine

what they could look like if the focus was on *you*, not the provider. Even if you're happy with everything, review some of your recent healthcare experiences as a thought experiment. What could have been better? More convenient? Imagine your doctor conducting a consumer survey or a focus group with yourself as a participant. What would some of your observations be? What changes for the better would you recommend? Now imagine that you can shop for those changes. Start thinking like a consumer with choices.

JOIN THE BROADER CONVERSATION

If you're managing a chronic condition like hypertension or diabetes, test out a few consumer-based websites, such as PatientsLikeMe, to see what kind of dialogue is going on.

Here again, we're talking mainly about acclimatization and familiarity, not drastic action for its own sake. We're certainly not suggesting you ignore your doctor's advice and abruptly follow the counsel of some fellow-sufferer patient on one of these websites. But you should at least be familiar with the kind of dialogue that is going on there, the types of issues and ideas that are being put forward. This could be a rich source of both inspiration and practical advice, and there is no downside to at least seeing what is going on and what folks are saying.

BE MORE PROACTIVE WITH YOUR PRIMARY CARE PROVIDER

This is a biggie. In the DefaultAging model, the entire relationship with your GP was on the doctor's terms—convenience of appointment (did it start on time), length of appointment, what the doctor did, questions they asked, and so on. You had little or no influence on the transaction, except to report how you were feeling. While this model is in retreat, it stubbornly persists within the medical community. Here are some shocking facts reported in an excellent article from the Patient Empowerment Network (yes, there is such a thing):

- The average visit lasts 15 minutes (according to Sir Muir Gray's book, in the United Kingdom it's only 8 minutes).
- Patients have an average of 23 seconds to state their concerns before the physician interrupts.
- Only 27% of physicians know the full range of their patient's concerns before they focus on a specific concern.
- Once they focus on that concern, the probability of returning to other concerns is only 8%.

Can you do anything to change this? The article offers a number of ideas, including:

- Be precise about the appointment: Why are you going, and how much time do *you* need? Write out your symptoms ahead of time, so you can be focused and accurate.
- If you're using a self-tracking device, download your data and bring it to the appointment.
- Bring a list (or even take photos) of all medications you're currently taking, including vitamins or supplements.
- Tell your doctor you want to make notes during the consultation.

- Don't be afraid to question what the doctor is saying if you don't understand or to ask if there are other options to the treatment.
- Get a copy of any test results.
- If there's a prescription, make sure you understand how and when it should be taken, what side effects you can expect, and how you'll know if it's working.
- Make notes when you get home. Include any test results and the billing. The notes may cause you to rethink parts of the visit or realize you need more information.
- Call the doctor and follow up—this redefines the visit as part of an ongoing process of healthcare management.
- Could your doctor be ageist? Ageism is an issue in medicine today, and, whether overt or subtle, it could be robbing you of better outcomes. If you are encountering ageism, it may be time to fire your physician (more on this in the Avoidance chapter).

CHECK IF YOUR HEALTH INSURANCE PROVIDER INCLUDES P4P

This is about changing your mindset so that you know more about what's going on and how all the pieces fit together when it comes to the management of your healthcare. Don't be afraid to call your insurance provider and ask if they offer some form of P4P or value modeling in their reimbursement program. If not, ask why. Are there other insurers you could switch to? If your insurance is mandated by your employer, what does HR think of the topic?

KEEP UP TO DATE WITH
NEW DEVELOPMENTS

In the field of healthcare, there are new ideas and improvements happening all the time. Check the Resources section at SuperAging.info.

DIET AND NUTRITION

Diet has *always* been a hot topic, and if anything, the advent of SuperAging has only increased the noise level. Every day seems to bring a new study, a new "expert" touting some "miracle" program.

Most of the action focuses on weight loss. This is an issue for all ages, and there is a program for every need, budget, attention span, level of patience, and intensity of desire. We have no interest in picking our way through that particular jungle.

There are a great many diets specifically designed to deal with chronic conditions—diets to promote heart health, to help control hypertension or diabetes, to reduce inflammation. In the Resources section at SuperAging.info, we provide a guide to the major disease-state associations along with information on specific diet plans. Obviously, if you're already on a good program, keep it up. In no way do we recommend abandoning what's working or what your doctor recommends.

That said, you don't necessarily even need a detailed diet or menu plan. There are a few critical principles you should be guided by and practices you can quickly incorporate into your daily routine.

MAKE DIET AND NUTRITION PART OF YOUR SUPERAGING PROGRAM

AS MUCH AS POSSIBLE, SHIFT TO A PLANT-BASED DIET

Of all the diets out there, the Blue Zone principle (or, if you want something more structured and formalized, the Mediterranean diet) has been shown to promote a longer life span. Harvard researchers, who in 2020 analyzed over 32 studies involving more than 700,000 people, found that people who got just 3% more of their total calories from plant protein (beans, nuts, whole grains) lowered their risk of premature death by 5%. Another study that same year found that shifting that same 3% of calorie intake from animal protein (meat, poultry, fish, dairy) to plant protein corresponded to a 10% decrease in death from any cause. What's more, researchers believe they understand why. A diet with a lot of fruits, legumes, beans, nuts, and seeds apparently extends the life of telomeres (see the Attitude chapter).

Does this mean all-vegan? No meat at all? There are many branches along the path, and you will have to choose what best suits your tastes and needs. A typical modification of all-vegan is to eat more fish but avoid red meat.

DRINK PLENTY OF WATER

This won't come as a surprise since virtually every diet or health program for every single age group includes this advice. But what's interesting in our SuperAging context is that hydration has been shown to be a key factor in longevity.

To be more accurate, it's dehydration that inhibits longevity. Dehydration causes more fatigue, a reduction in mental energy, and less efficient digestion. "Dehydration is probably the number one disease," says Dr. Will Simmons, a Florida-based physical therapist we interviewed. "If people were hydrated properly, their bodies would function better, their immune systems would do their jobs better."

If you're wondering how much water, Dr. Simmons says you should be drinking "regularly" throughout the day. An easy-to-remember rule is 8 × 8: eight glasses of water, each glass being eight fluid ounces. Be aware that there are some risks associated with drinking too much water, particularly if you have kidney issues. It's wise to check with your doctor.

PRACTICE PORTION CONTROL

A good way to eat in moderation is to control portion sizes. People usually eat everything they dish out, so if you have smaller portions, you'll automatically be reducing the tendency to overeat. Numerous guides show how to do this, offering all kinds of refinements based on your weight and your food preferences. But without making it too complicated, here are a few simple steps to get you started:

Use smaller plates. Numerous studies have shown that people who use bigger dishes eat more, and are often unaware of how big their portions are.

Use the plate or bowl itself to mark out the portion. A quick guide is to use half the plate for vegetables or a salad, a quarter for protein (meat, fish, poultry, eggs), and a quarter for carbs (whole grains, starchy vegetables). If you're also having butter or cheese, use only half a tablespoon.

Use your hands to determine portion size. An alternative formula involves using your hands. For the main protein dish, for example, use one palm-sized serving for a woman and two for a man. For salads and veggies, two fist-sized portions for a woman and one for a man.

DRINK ALCOHOL, BUT IN MODERATION

A feature of the Blue Zone program was that the centenarians drank one to two glasses of red wine per day. We all know that excessive alcohol drinking can be bad for you, but it appears that drinking in moderation can be good and even promote longevity. One study found that both men and women who averaged one alcoholic beverage per day had a better chance of reaching age 90 than either heavy drinkers or outright abstainers. More specifically, other studies show that moderate alcohol drinkers have a lower risk of cardiovascular problems than nondrinkers.

Is there a reason?

Alcohol appears to affect the mTOR pathway. mTOR (mechanistic target of rapamycin) is a protein enzyme that regulates cell growth, and its suppression can slow the aging of cells. Alcohol has positive health benefits too. It can lower the risk of atherosclerosis (hardening of the arteries) by increasing HDL (good cholesterol) levels. A moderate amount of alcohol also exerts an anti-inflammatory effect, though the opposite is true if you drink too much. Wine in particular has high amounts of polyphenols, which help protect against cardiovascular disease and some cancers. Red wine also contains resveratrol, a compound that reduces risk of coronary heart disease and cancer. Whiskey also contains polyphenol compounds.

CONSIDER THE BENEFITS OF FASTING

Intermittent fasting has been shown to promote healthy aging. This seems to have to do with mitochondria, the energy-producing structures in cells. They change their shape according to energy demand, but their capacity to do this declines with age. Research indicates that calorie restriction can help maintain the mitochondria in their "youthful" state, which contributes to an increase in life span.

This dynamic was originally discovered in lab tests with earthworms, but numerous other studies have confirmed the longevity-promoting effects of intermittent fasting. It reduces oxidative stress (the imbalance between free radicals and antioxidants) and protects against type 2 diabetes, hypertension, and cardiovascular disease. Other studies suggest it can reduce the risk of asthma, arthritis, and even Alzheimer's.

There are several recognized variations:

Time-restricted feeding (TRF): You eat only during a certain window (for example, 10:00 a.m.–6:00 p.m.) and then have an extended fast overnight.

Alternate-day fasting: You fast or restrict your calorie intake every second day.

Intermittent 5:2: You fast two days a week and eat normally on the other five.

For obvious reasons, you must check with your doctor before you get into any of this. TRF is clearly the easiest first step: it's not a particularly big stretch to go from a "last meal of the day" at 6:00 p.m. to a "first meal of the day" at 10:00 the next morning. Not eating at all for a whole day is a much bigger step. But the advantages of an intermittent fasting program are quite compelling.

FITNESS AND EXERCISE

Just as with diet and nutrition, the field of fitness and exercise is jam-packed with advice. There are books, blogs, instructional videos, and apps, plus an enormous range of exercise facilities offering various levels of complexity and expense.

You'll find some of our favorite books and websites listed in the Resources section at SuperAging.info, but for the purposes of this chapter we want to highlight a few important examples of fresh thinking, issues you should be aware of, and relatively simple steps you can take right away to either begin an exercise program or incorporate into what you're doing already. The focus here is on longevity, not necessarily weight loss or sports training. If you're already engaged in a program and you're happy with how it's going, keep it up! Also, be sure to check with your doctor before undertaking anything new.

One common barrier to starting an exercise program is the misconception that it may be too late to do you any good. The DefaultAging world seemed to be divided into people who exercised regularly since their youth and those who never did anything. As the years went by, this second group never quite got going, and it became easier to stay idle by convincing yourself that the window of opportunity had passed. Okay, maybe you wanted to be careful about what you ate, but really, what could working out accomplish at this stage of the game, in your 60s, 70s, or 80s?

The research shows that it can accomplish plenty.

A landmark study over a decade ago took 24 people between 91 and 96 years old and divided them into an exercise group and a control group. The exercise group underwent a 12-week program of twice-a-week workouts, combining strength training and balance improvement exercises. Results: increased walking speed, improvement in balance (and significant reduction in the incidence of falls), and improved muscle power and mass in the lower limbs. "The study has shown that power training can be perfectly applied to the elderly with frailty," the researchers reported.

Another study, which was described in an article on Healthline entitled "Why It's Never Too Late to Start Exercising," compared men in their 70s and 80s who had never exercised regularly to master athletes of the same age—those who had worked out all their lives and still competed in their sports. Both groups went through a single weight-training session on an exercise machine. Researchers gave an isotope tracer before the workout so as to track how proteins were developing in their muscles, and took muscle biopsies from both groups before and after. The hypothesis was that the master athletes would be much better able to build muscle during exercise, but the results showed that both groups had an equal capacity to do that. According to lead researcher Leigh Breen, "Our study clearly shows that it doesn't matter if you haven't been a regular exerciser throughout your life; you can still derive benefit from exercise whenever you start."

MAKE FITNESS AND EXERCISE PART OF YOUR SUPERAGING PROGRAM

WALK, STRENGTH TRAIN, AND SQUAT

One barrier to doing exercise is the perception that it's complex, time-consuming, and costly. You need equipment, and if you don't have enough room in your home, that means joining a gym or maybe even getting a personal trainer. The misperceptions quickly accumulate until "exercise" becomes a whole separate world, difficult to access. While exercise may indeed be complex or costly if the goal is to become a bodybuilder, that's not our goal here.

Recent advice is shifting in the direction of simplicity, especially for healthy longevity as opposed to high-level athletic performance. You don't need a gym or a personal trainer. You can incorporate exercise easily into a convenient daily routine.

For example, the simple act of walking is now seen as a powerful contributor to longevity. A study in the *Journal of the American Geriatrics Society* found that people over the age of 65 could lower their risk of cardiovascular disease with about four hours of walking per week, an average of only half an hour a day. Another study published in the *Journal of Alzheimer's Disease* found that a brisk half-hour walk stimulated blood flow to the brain and contributed to improved performance, including memory function. Most recently, a study published in *JAMA Internal Medicine* found that adding as few as 10 minutes of walking to the normal daily routine could lower the risk of premature death. In fact, they calculated that if everyone did that, it could save over 100,000 Americans from premature death every year!

Walking is an ideal form of exercise for SuperAgers because it's low-impact, safe, convenient, and free. You can start right away, and gradually build up distance and speed. The health benefits, as noted by numerous research studies, are many: stronger bones and muscles, improved endurance, higher energy level, better cardiovascular fitness, better balance and coordination, and even a stronger immune system.

But not all walking is equal. Studies also show that brisk walking is much better than slow ambling. A 2021 study at the University of Leicester found that slow walkers were four times more likely to die from severe cases of COVID than brisk walkers.

According to the *Daily Mail*, lead researcher Tom Yates indicated that fast walkers can have up to 20 more years of life, perhaps due to the fact that doing so strengthens the cardiovascular system and improves the body's capacity to utilize oxygen. This insight is supported by plenty of other research, like a 2015 study in the *American Journal of Clinical Nutrition*, which found that a brisk 20-minute walk every day could reduce risk of death by more than 30%.

But how do you know what speed is right? One good rule of thumb that we like is this: you should be able to carry on a conversation, but you're moving too quickly to be able to sing a song.

Remember, too, that speed is only one variable. You can also put more power and physical exertion into the walk. One increasingly popular method is to use walking poles. Pole walking burns 46% more calories than regular walking because you're working your upper body as well as your legs. But the support from the poles means it actually feels easier. The best poles are the so-called Nordic-style poles, which have thumb-hole hand straps, a streamlined shape, and full-size rubber feet. With Nordic poles, you are using as much as 90% of your body muscles as you walk—significantly better results than trekking or strapless walking sticks.

We talked about Nordic walking poles with Bill VanGorder, COO of CARP (Canadian Association of Retired Persons), who is a colleague of David's. He added a side business as a dealer in Nordic poles (a perfect SuperAger response to conventional retirement, as you'll see in the chapter on Accomplishment!). "The beauty is that because you're working the upper body as well, you're burning these extra calories without needing to speed up your walking pace," Bill explained. "It improves your cardio, your balance, and your muscle strength all at the same time."

Walking, especially with Nordic poles, is easy to implement, does not interfere with what you may already be doing, and research insights show it is more than worthwhile. But other expert opinions insist that walking alone isn't enough. You also need to counter the loss of muscle mass that accompanies aging, and for that you need some form of resistance training as well.

Physical therapist Will Simmons was particularly outspoken on this. "When older people think about exercise," he told us, "for them, a lot of it is walking. It's convenient, it doesn't cost much, you're moving; it's been pushed by the media—get up, get off the couch, move around. But it doesn't go far enough."

Your exercise program must also include strength training, he says, preferably two to three times a week. The methods can be quite varied, using weights, resistance bands, or apparatus in a gym or at home. In fact, he's happy if you mix and match, but the important point is that you must include some form of strength training in your program.

Luckily, there are a huge number of books, blogs, and YouTube videos that offer programs tailored to older people, and our favorites are listed in the Resources section at SuperAging.info. The good news is that this need not be a big, complex program; important benefits can be gained in as little as 20 minutes of resistance work, three or four times a week. Nor do you need to invest in a lot of complex equipment. There are many programs that employ only dumbbells or resistance bands, which are inexpensive. You can do everything at home.

The last exercise you might consider requires no equipment at all and confers many benefits. We're talking about squats. Squats are easy to do: you stand up, hold your hands in front of your heart (or hold a dumbbell), then bend at the knees, sitting back on your heels and hips until your thighs are parallel to the ground. Pay special attention to your knees so they don't extend over your toes. Go down as low as you can, then rise back up again. Work your way up to enough reps that you're spending about three minutes (five is better), and do this three times a week.

Squats combine more benefits in one simple move than probably any other single form of exercise. First, you're involving (and thus strengthening) a lot of different muscles—rear, quads, calves, hamstrings, hips. Second, you're alternately increasing and decreasing the blood flow to the brain, which can have the effect of stimulating and nourishing the hippocampus, the brain's memory center. Get squatting!

STRENGTHEN YOUR CORE

Try this simple test. Stand on one foot (use either foot). Place the front of your free foot around the back of the foot that's on the floor. The free foot doesn't need to be high off the floor; it can just tuck in above and behind the ankle of the foot on the floor—the important point is that only one foot is touching the floor. Hold your arms to the sides and look straight ahead. Hold the position for 10 seconds. If you can't do it at first, give yourself three tries.

Simple, right? But an international team of researchers believe that success or failure could be a predictor of longevity.

They looked at data collected between 2009 and 2020 on 1,700 Brazilians, aged 51 to 75. Allowing for differences in age, sex, and underlying health conditions, those who failed the balance test had an 84% higher risk of death—from any cause—in the subsequent decade.

About one in five failed the test. Not surprisingly, failure rates increased with age, ranging from 5% failure in the youngest group to 54% for the oldest (aged 71–75). On an average seven-year follow-up, about 7% of participants had died, with a heavier concentration among those who failed the test.

Since deaths were from all causes, not just falls and injuries, the underlying mechanics aren't completely clear. We don't know for sure the underlying physical or biological reasons that failure on the balance test would be a sign of higher future risk of death. But even if we deliberately narrowed our focus to balance only as a protection against falling and being injured, there are serious life and death implications. Falls are a major public health issue for the older population. United States statistics are particularly revealing:

- About 36 million falls are reported among older adults every year, resulting in more than 32,000 deaths.
- Over three million older adults are treated in emergency departments for a fall injury each year.
- Over 300,000 older people are hospitalized for hip fractures every year, of which more than 90% are caused by falling.

Fortunately, this is a topic gaining more attention, and there are numerous relatively simple exercises you can do to strengthen your core and reduce the risk of falling. There are some very simple core-strengthening exercises, like pelvic tilts and bridges, that are easy to learn. Check the Resources section at SuperAging.info for more.

IMPROVE YOUR FLEXIBILITY

Aging can bring with it a decrease in the elasticity of your muscles, leading to a smaller range of motion in your shoulders, spine, and hips, compounded by more aches and pains. Stretching is the best way to counter this. It is easy (some stretches can be performed while sitting in a chair), can be gentle, and works wonders if you're consistent.

Regular stretching can improve your circulation, reduce your risk of joint and muscle pain, help you relax, and increase that range of motion (making all your other exercises more effective). You could look into tai chi for balance and yoga or Pilates for flexibility. But even if you don't start a full program (just yet), only 10 minutes a day of simple stretching exercises will work wonders.

Check the Resources section at SuperAging.info for more.

PRACTICE GOOD SLEEP HABITS

We all probably believe, in a general sort of way, that "getting a good night's sleep" is a Good Thing. But does it link specifically to aging and longevity?

The research is clear. Sleep deprivation produces many harmful effects on all ages, but there are particular implications for older people. A 2021 study found a connection between sleep problems and increased risk for dementia. On the positive side, a 2014 study found that the oldest individuals (aged 85–105) had more regular sleep patterns than younger individuals, and researchers concluded that "human longevity is associated with regular sleep patterns."

We were surprised (perhaps we shouldn't have been) to find there is a lot of activity around trying to develop better approaches to sleep or at least systematizing the approaches so that they are not just vague tips. There are a lot of new treatments and products that can help.

Cognitive behavioral therapy (CBT) is at work in this field, and Stanford University has developed a whole tool kit to cope with insomnia. The techniques include stimulus control (keeping a consistent wake-up time and only getting into bed when sleepy), reducing time spent lying awake, employing stress management and relaxation techniques, and seeking professional help to shift your circadian clock through techniques such as light exposure therapy.

This last item is particularly interesting. Researchers discovered that ultrashort bursts of light directed at a person's closed eyes while they were sleeping were very effective at shifting the time they start getting sleepy. This short-flash method involves wearing a sleep mask that emits the bright flashes and only wakes people who are particularly sensitive to light. This has already been turned into a product.

There are also numerous sleep apps, and even an online course developed by the Cleveland Clinic. The six-week course uses CBT techniques to help you identify and then reframe thoughts and behaviors that are interfering with proper sleep. Check the Resources at SuperAging.info for more information.

Don't ignore simpler steps either. A lighter meal at night or a walk after dinner can also promote better sleep.

CONSIDER TEAM SPORTS

Here's another less obvious trend you may not be aware of: getting your exercise in the form of team sports. Many SuperAgers are doing this, and it conveys benefits beyond what exercise alone can accomplish. The big one, of course, is that team sports create a social network and reduce feelings of isolation or loneliness. They also enhance self-esteem and create an emotionally satisfying set of goals (teamwork, winning competitions) that contribute to better mental health.

This isn't just conjecture. A 2019 study, which analyzed 30 other studies, found that older participants in team sports reported better health, feeling part of a community (including more opportunities to develop new relationships), strong feelings of achievement, and even more occasions to travel. Another study reported very positive attitudes on the part of competitive sports participants. "I'm out here, and I can do this!" was the typical comment. They identified themselves as different from the stereotypical older person who is frail and dependent (the DefaultAger, if you will). They saw team competition, even friendly competition, as an opportunity to push themselves and demonstrate that they still had strength and confidence. Many saw it as a deliberate and active response to the aging process— they were consciously aware of being SuperAgers! They felt a sense of empowerment and pride.

Just how much this is happening can be shown by a small sample of Canadian statistics, courtesy of Vividata, the best consumer database we know of. Here is how many Canadians over the age of 65 took part in competitive or team sports in 2022:

- Downhill skiing—186,000
- Cross-country skiing—193,000
- Skating—229,000
- Basketball—75,000
- Football—45,000
- Volleyball—81,000
- Ice hockey—143,000
- Curling—100,000

It's happening. There are dozens of associations that promote team sports for SuperAgers. If you'd like to get involved, check the Resources section at SuperAging.info for some ideas.

LEARN ABOUT EXERCISE SNACKS

This is a new idea, which is gaining a lot of popularity in the physical fitness world, derived from the Blue Zones example. Blue Zone centenarians don't work out in a separate and extended time block; rather, they keep moving and have mini-bursts of extra physical activity all day long. The food metaphor works perfectly—instead of a longer exercise "meal" (30–45 minutes in the gym), you "snack" on small increments of exercise throughout the entire day.

Each snack is typically only a few minutes long, and most snackers do it at least four or five times a day.

And it works! Many studies have shown that small breaks of exercise throughout the day can be very good for your health. In one large study involving more than 44,000 men and women, researchers found that as little as 11 minutes of activity for otherwise sedentary people could reduce the risk of early death. Previous wisdom was that it required an hour a day to create cardiovascular improvement.

New research also suggests that staying sedentary may change the behavior of the gene responsible for producing an enzyme that breaks down fat. Dr. Martin Gibala, professor of kinesiology at McMaster University, Hamilton, Canada, explained the dynamics in an article on the Blue Zones website. Basically, being active, even in short bursts, speeds up your metabolism.

What kinds of activities constitute exercise snacks? Here's an easy, equipment-free set you can do anywhere, cited by Dr. Gibala:

- Warm-up: easy jumping jacks—60 seconds
- Squat followed by jumping in the air (essentially a burpee without the push-up)—60 seconds
- High-kneed running in place—60 seconds

- Jump in the air and land in a squat position, alternate legs (split squat jump)—60 seconds

You could do all of these and intersperse them with a 60-second rest in which you walked in place. The pattern would be: warm-up | squat | rest | high-kneed running | rest | split squat | rest | high-kneed running | rest | squat | rest. This would add up to an 11-minute workout, which can easily be done (perhaps more than once) during a typical day.

For those who can't run or jump, possibly because of ankle or knee issues, there are some very effective workouts, some as short as five minutes, that involve walking in place (standing or even sitting) punctuated by straight-ahead fist punches, diagonal punches or reaches, bicep curls, and elbow lifts. We link to some of them at SuperAging.info.

KNOW YOUR NUMBERS

You are probably already familiar with fitness trackers, like the Fitbit, Apple Watch, or Samsung Galaxy watch. These wearable devices monitor physical activity like the number of steps you take or the number of calories you burn, and record associated measurements like heart rate. But you may be surprised to learn how advanced the wearable industry has become. You now have an unparalleled ability to know your numbers for a lot more than just the immediate measurements associated with exercise or other physical activity.

Some wearables can now monitor your health 24/7, not just in response to exercise. Heart rate monitors are now standard on many smart watches, and models are appearing on the market that can detect abnormalities like atrial fibrillation, when the heart quivers instead of beats, which is a major cause of stroke.

Sleep patterns can also be monitored. Apple's Series 7 model checks blood oxygen levels and sleep patterns, detects falls and can automatically call 911 if it senses you're not moving, and even allows you to take an electrocardiogram. Not surprisingly, usage is exploding. Over 300 million people already use some form of wearable, and in 2020 the world market was worth over $40 billion.

And the future is more exciting still. New technology based on harvesting energy from the surrounding area may reduce or eliminate the need to change batteries. Single-topic monitoring (like blood glucose levels) is already possible with subcutaneous sensors. And why does "wearable" have to apply only to a watch? Smart clothing is already here: there are smart socks that can detect which parts of your feet are receiving too much pressure when you run and smart sleepwear that absorbs heat from your body and releases infrared light to boost sleep quality and muscle recovery.

The data doesn't have to be only for you either. Wearables can and do send key information to healthcare providers in real time, alerting them to changes in your physical condition that may require intervention. In the DefaultAging model, your doctor took your blood pressure during a checkup, but neither you nor they knew the numbers in between visits. Then small, portable blood pressure cuffs came on the market, enabling you to run your own tests. But you had to phone or email the results to your doctor. With wearables, the data can be sent constantly, and AI can analyze it against predetermined benchmarks or diagnoses, enabling a doctor, nurse, or other provider to be instantly responsive to a sudden change or need.

Bottom line: It's never been more possible to know your numbers and to know them across a much wider range of health topics. It's never been more possible to leverage that knowledge in real time to produce more timely responses and better outcomes. Knowing your numbers enables SuperAgers to take more control.

A Better Relationship with Your Body: Tips from Physical Therapist Will Simmons, DPT

Dr. Simmons offers a refreshing and inspiring view of longevity: the key is to consider the body as a whole. "My first job," he explains, "is to help my patients have a better relationship with their body."

The first priority is oxygen. "This means you've got to learn how to breathe with your diaphragm. Teaching my patients how to breathe is a big part of physical therapy."

The diaphragm is the main muscle of respiration; it separates the thoracic cavity from the abdominal cavity. Involving your diaphragm in breathing, as opposed to just using your lungs, increases the volume of air coming into the system and improves the efficiency of the exchange of gases—oxygen coming in, carbon dioxide going out. This decreases blood pressure and heart rate, improving circulation and reducing the workload on the heart.

"Learning how to breathe with the diaphragm," he points out, "is one of the reasons you see so much longevity in some of the Eastern practices—the yogis, the Buddhist monks, the Taoist masters. It's because a key focus of theirs is diaphragmatic breathing."

If oxygen is foundational, so is water. As we noted previously, Dr. Simmons wants us to drink water regularly all day long.

He's also worried about food, specifically, sugar. "We've got our bodies stranded in deserts of sugar and inactivity and stasis and stress, and it makes it that much harder to let the body heal and reach our full potential."

His biggest theme is that our body is designed to heal more and last longer than we're letting it. Whether it's improper breathing, not enough water, or too much sugar in our diets, these things are interfering with the natural ability of the body to thrive. We're impeding what should be happening naturally. If we don't deal with these issues, then no workout program can save the day.

And even when it comes to workout programs, Dr. Simmons starts with foundational issues before offering specific workout plans. He believes there is a lot of confusion about exercise as it applies to longevity. "In general, men think all they have to do is lift weights," he says. "Women think what they need to focus on is cardio and flexibility. But a woman's body is made to carry a child and has more mobility and flexibility already because of its bone structure. What it needs is more strength, more resistance work. A man's body, on the other hand, where it's easier to pack on more dense muscle fiber, needs more of the flexibility and mobility to take some of the stress off the joints."

He's talking about a rebalancing, of course, not a complete flip-flop. The end result must be to include both resistance work and exercises to promote mobility and flexibility.

But here again, Dr. Simmons has an overview that comes before determining the list of individual exercises. He believes we must start by learning how to move properly. "Healthy physical function means learning how to move our body in a different plane—forward, backward, side to side, and rotationally with precision," he told us, "and then incorporating functional strengthening into that." He recommends that everyone go to a physical therapist for an audit of how you move now and how to improve. "Go once a week for four weeks," he said, "and learn what you can." Improving the way you move, which includes posture and core strengthening, will then positively affect all the forms of exercise you choose to do.

Dr. Simmons's approach is refreshing and creative because he doesn't just jump to a list of specific exercises. He wants the pieces to fit together into a holistic strategy, one that addresses the foundational issues. If the underlying fundamentals are there—the attention to breathing, water intake, diet, proper form of body movement—then the specific exercises can be many, and mix 'n' match is great.

Dr. Simmons has a great video on how to breathe properly, and you'll find a link to that at SuperAging.info.

BRAIN HEALTH

Mental fitness, or brain health, is the last topic for Activity, and in some ways, it is the most elusive.

There is a great deal of misunderstanding—and outright misinformation—about what brain health actually is and whether you can do anything about it. All discussions seem to be overlaid by the dreaded specter of dementia and Alzheimer's disease, but among the general public there is a widespread lack of knowledge about what these conditions are in the first place, what causes them, and what can be done to mitigate them. The fear and sense of helplessness is so great that many people fail to report memory loss issues because they just don't want to know they are on the road to dementia and Alzheimer's.

In this sense, brain health is a couple of decades behind physical health when it comes to accepting a certain degree of decline and not panicking about it, and when it comes to believing in the possibilities of prevention or mitigation. Even people who view aging with optimism understand that the body may slow down and that there may be new aches and pains, but this isn't necessarily the end of the world. Even people who don't work out believe—if only because they see so many examples of people who do—that you can stay fit for longer if you exercise. But when it comes to the brain, things get mysterious and myths prevail. Among the most common myths about brain health:

Dementia and Alzheimer's are the same thing. Alzheimer's is a type of dementia caused by a speeding up of normal aging in the brain. Vascular dementia is caused by a lack of oxygen reaching the brain, which in turn causes cell damage. Lewy body dementia is caused by a buildup of the protein for which it is named; these proteins are also associated with Parkinson's disease. The fourth main type is frontotemporal dementia, caused by damage to the brain cells in the frontal and temporal lobes, where problem-solving, recognition, and behavior are controlled. It's true that Alzheimer's is the most common form, accounting for about 60% of all diagnoses.

Dementia is inevitable. Dementia itself is not necessarily a normal part of aging. In fact, only about one in seven adults over the age of 70 have some form of dementia.

Dementia is a "disease" that you may or may not "get," especially as you age. Not true. Dementia is a syndrome—that is, the result of a complex of symptoms and not one condition. There are risk factors that have been identified; there are preventive measures that can be taken.

It's true that some factors may involve hereditary influences, but SuperAgers should approach brain health the same way they approach body health: it's something that requires and deserves proactive measures, and it can be managed so as to reduce or delay the most harmful effects.

That management process should start by recognizing that brain health is an important part of overall health. We were guided into this understanding by Dr. Allison Sekuler, vice president of research at Baycrest Health Sciences in Toronto, one of the foremost brain health research centers in the world.

There are aspects of physical health and well-being, she told us, that represent known risk factors for dementia, such as vision and hearing loss. Both increase the cognitive load on the brain: the brain has to work harder to see and hear, which diverts its resources from other processes like memory. Studies have shown, for example, that people who have problems hearing or identifying speech against an overall background of noise are more likely to develop dementia than people with normal hearing. This makes it very important for SuperAgers to frequently test eyesight and hearing, and to take remedial action that is usually easily available. It's not a matter of naturally reducing hearing or vision loss, which can certainly occur with aging, but mitigating it so that it does not produce increased workload on the brain.

Another risk factor is lack of sleep. While the mechanics are still not entirely understood or agreed upon, one theory is that when we sleep, the brain flushes out some of the day's natural accumulation of beta-amyloid, a protein associated with Alzheimer's. If you don't get enough sleep, the beta-amyloids build up. Whatever the underlying biochemistry, the research confirms a direct correlation: one study found that people in their 50s and 60s who got six hours of sleep or less were 30% more likely to be diagnosed with dementia than those who got seven hours or more.

Another important issue that SuperAgers should pay attention to is loneliness. The correlation between loneliness and dementia risk has been well established, though the underlying causes are not crystal clear. Studies show that loneliness is associated with a 26% higher risk of dementia. One possible reason is that lonely people have poorer overall health and health behaviors—less exercise, lack of sleep, and more depression, which is itself a risk factor. Some research suggests that lonely people have higher levels of beta-amyloid.

"We know social interaction is important," Dr. Sekuler told us. "We know stress reduction is important, and there is a relationship between loneliness and stress."

In the upcoming chapter on Attachment, we'll deal more extensively with the problems of social isolation and the remedies, including the rapid development of tech solutions that are particularly effective in remote communities. Dr. Sekuler mentioned there's a lot of research going on to learn more, at the biological level, about the differences between in-person contact and digital contact. On the one hand, digital contact can be scalable and can reach people with poor or nonexistent support networks; on the other hand, in-person contact affects the brain in a way that digital connections can't duplicate. "Going forward," she said, "I think we'll see a mix of virtual and personal, tailored to the individual's needs and activities."

MAKE BRAIN HEALTH PART OF YOUR SUPERAGING PROGRAM

TRY NEW THINGS

"The brain is a novelty-seeking device," Dr. Sekuler says. "If you're perseverating on one idea—which is something that can happen with aging—you end up with the inability to change from one thing to the next. The more you can practice enabling yourself to move from one kind of idea to another, the better."

The key is to offer variety. Many people gravitate to brain games and puzzles, but it's important not to limit yourself to things you've already mastered. You can keep doing those things for pure recreational enjoyment, of course, but for better brain health, also tackle new types of puzzles or games that you're not familiar with.

Learning a new language is another good approach. In fact, learning a new anything—art making, singing, improv—will work.

SLEEP WELL

As noted previously, there is a connection between lack of sleep and heightened risk for dementia. One study showed that compared to people getting seven hours' sleep, people getting fewer hours each night are 30% more likely to be diagnosed with dementia. Some researchers believe it could be due to a buildup of beta-amyloid fluid, a metabolic waste that is cleared out of the brain during sleep.

Whatever the underlying causes, it's clear that sleep deprivation increases your risk and better sleep reduces it. Go back and check the section on sleep habits earlier in this chapter and make sure you're following the recommendations.

BE AWARE OF BRAIN FOODS

There is no single magic food that will prevent cognitive decline. But knowing how much is riding on a strong performance by your heart and blood vessels, you can identify which foods are particularly valuable in promoting brain health:

- Green, leafy vegetables like kale, spinach, and broccoli are loaded with critical nutrients like vitamin K, which helps make proteins needed for the building of bones, and beta carotene, which converts into vitamin A and then plays an important role in cell growth and maintaining the health of the heart, lungs, and kidneys.

- Fatty fish contribute omega-3 fatty acids, which have been linked to lower levels of beta-amyloid.
- Tea and coffee—it's true. Research has shown a statistical correlation between caffeine consumption and better memory.
- Berries contribute flavonoids, the natural pigments that give berries their color. A Harvard study showed that women who had two or more servings of berries a week delayed memory decline by as much as two and a half years.
- Walnuts contribute alpha-linolenic acid, which has been linked to lower blood pressure.

UNDERSTAND HOW PHYSICAL ACTIVITY HELPS THE BRAIN

As we've already seen, physical activity promotes better health and longevity in many ways, but it's good to know there are some important direct benefits for your brain. Physical activity promotes increased oxygen flow (reread Dr. Will Simmons's advice about learning to breathe with your diaphragm) and the growth of new nerve cells and synapses in the brain. It also lowers blood pressure and reduces stress, both of which are negative factors that increase the risk of dementia.

NURTURE SOCIAL CONNECTIONS

As Dr. Sekuler pointed out, loneliness and isolation increase the risk of dementia. So nurturing social connections becomes a big issue in the promotion of brain health. It's such a big topic, in fact, that it makes up one of our seven *A*'s of SuperAging. The chapter on Attachment will present all the essential information you need on why this matters and what to do about it.

Keeping Your Brain Active: A Multidirectional Approach from Dr. Allison Sekuler

Dr. Allison Sekuler is one of the foremost brain health scientists and researchers in North America. So we weren't surprised to see her formidable credentials: vice president of research at Baycrest Health Sciences and managing director of its Centre for Aging and Brain Health Innovation, managing director and senior scientist at the Rotman Research Institute, professor at the University of Toronto and McMaster University, and . . . drummer?

Seriously?

Yes. So seriously, in fact, that she's looking forward to a second career as a drummer once she retires from science and medicine. Her interest in drumming is really a matter of her practicing what she preaches by bringing diversity to her brain activity.

"I'm a big fan of drumming," she told us, "because each limb is doing something different, and you also have to be listening to the entire band. You have to be listening to what each instrument is doing so you can respond as part of a musical conversation. It's brain training."

Dr. Sekuler likes music in general as a brain-stimulating activity, whether learning to play a new instrument or just exploring as a listener. One study found that musicians were 64% less likely to develop mild cognitive impairment than nonmusicians, while frequent musicians (professional or not) had 80% higher chances of being in the top cognitive decile.

Two keys to brain health, as we've seen, are challenge and variety. Music by its very nature delivers on both, whether new skills to be mastered, a new piece to be learned or understood at a new or deeper level, or entirely new formats to be explored.

There's also the aspect of moving in new directions. This goes beyond brain health alone and becomes a key driver of the whole SuperAging program; the upcoming chapter on Accomplishment explores this in detail.

For Dr. Sekuler, that new direction will be a second career as a professional drummer. Why not? "Whatever brings you joy," she told us, "whatever you're excited by, that's what you should keep doing."

5

ACCOMPLISHMENT

We come now to our fourth *A*, Accomplishment. In the context of SuperAging, it means viewing the post-65 phase of life not as a period of retreat and disengagement but as an extended and positive opportunity to continue to grow and achieve goals. Specifically, life past 65 could include:

- A continuation of past employment rather than retirement on schedule (per the DefaultAging model).
- A replacement of past employment with some new full- or part-time employment.
- The acquisition or creation of a new business.
- A commitment to nonmonetary employment, such as volunteering, community service, or some other form of social activism.
- A return to full- or part-time education, such as a university degree, especially where such a pursuit was not possible in the younger years.

- The development of entirely new skills, such as learning a new language.
- The improvement of family relationships (often with the help of therapy or training).
- The pursuit of new contacts and social networks.

All of these are only marginally present, if they exist at all, in the DefaultAging model. That's because the model is driven, more than anything else, by the concept of retirement, where on a certain date, you cease employment and begin to collect a payout—some combination of savings and investments, private pension, and government pension—which provides you with enough money to live out the remaining years of your life. And it's a short period, usually no more than 10–15 years or so.

That's the model. And in the DefaultAging world, it worked. Given that you entered the job market in your young 20s, you had 40-some years in which to accumulate the funds and the pension entitlement for that last phase of life. You can see right away that the model leaves little or no room for Accomplishment to be much of a factor. The most important (or certainly, the most time-consuming) thing you've accomplished—your full-time job—abruptly ceases altogether, and you're not set up to do some new Big Thing. And in any case, you're going to be dead in 10 years or so, so what is there left to accomplish in such a short period of time?

Not only that, but the situation you're now in—retirement—implies a withdrawal from life, a curtailment of activity. And far from being an unattractive condition to be in, it's portrayed in warm and sentimental terms, particularly in advertising. The imagery is rich in non-activities like sitting on the beach and enjoying the view of the ocean, puttering around on the golf course or in the garden, taking a cruise. Idleness becomes the whole point: you deserve it, you've earned it, and at last you can finally afford it! Forget about accomplishing anything, you're barely *doing* anything. But that's wonderful. That's your well-deserved reward. Why else were you working so hard for all those years?

But today, that model is disappearing right before our eyes.

SuperAgers view the post-65 period of life as a time not just for the continuation of living, but for the continuation of accomplishing. The big reason, once again, is longevity. If you now have 20–30 years of post-65 life ahead of you, the notion of staying idle for that length of time and giving up on the possibility of accomplishing new things becomes increasingly absurd. (And, as we will see, financially difficult to the point of impossible.)

The pursuit of Accomplishment is revolutionizing our entire society. And at the individual level it is, in and of itself, a force for extending life even further. Accomplishment, promoted by longevity, produces even further longevity.

Let's start by looking at the most obvious manifestation of all this: employment and the evolution of retirement.

EMPLOYMENT

What do you do for a living? How much money do you make? In the DefaultAging world, the answers to these questions went a long way to characterizing your entire identity. The answers also set up your specific version of retirement—by definition, the job you held was what you were retiring *from.*

Retirement at 65 continues to be used as a benchmark; from public policy documents to news stories, we keep reading about how many Baby Boomers are reaching "the age of retirement," as if this was some kind of absolute standard even if it was being followed any longer.

And make no mistake—it is not being followed.

In the United States, United Kingdom, and Canada, the percentage of those over the age of 65 who are still in the workforce increases every year, showing a growth rate in contrast to younger workers, whose percentage of workforce participation is flat or declining. The number of Americans over the age of 75 who are still in the workforce is expected to double over the next 10 years.

Not surprisingly, then, numerous polls show that more and more older workers expect to keep working well beyond age 65. For example, a poll reported by AARP in 2017 indicated that half of all workers aged 60 and over said they planned to keep working until at least 70, and 20% said they didn't think they would *ever* retire. In a United Kingdom poll, more than half of 60-year-olds said they would need to keep working beyond the state pension retirement age. There are many other examples with similar findings.

There are three main factors driving all this:

1. **The underfunding of traditional retirement.**
   People haven't accumulated or simply can't accumulate enough savings and future pension entitlements to fund a post-65 life span of 20–30 years. They need to keep working because they need to keep generating income.
2. **The generational characteristics and attitudes of Baby Boomers, who now dominate the post-65 age group.** The original "Me" generation sees no reason to exit the stage.
3. **The realization that society needs more older workers to make up for shortfalls in the percentage of younger workers.** Collapsing birth rates compounded by dramatically greater longevity means that younger people represent a decreasing share of

the workforce. This in turn produces conditions that encourage older workers to keep working.

THE UNDERFUNDING OF TRADITIONAL RETIREMENT

It's one thing to retire and need money to pay for 10–15 more years of post-65 life. But 20–30 years?

The ugly truth: no way. Especially given the average savings that the older generations have in fact accumulated. The latest research shows the same inadequate level of retirement kitty for Baby Boomers in the United States, United Kingdom, and Canada: an average of somewhere in the $150,000 to $200,000 range. Even at double today's interest rates, this would throw off an annual investment income of only $12,000 to $15,000 (pretax). Add Social Security or Canada Pension or the UK State Pension, and you're looking at another $10,000 to $15,000 per annum. So you have maybe $30,000 (again, pretax) to live on, and you have to do that for 20–30 years.

Don't forget, we're using an average here. The statistics in all three countries also show that 20%–25% of Baby Boomers have retirement savings significantly less than the average, or none at all.

Where's the money going to come from?

Clearly, you have to keep earning an income. We'll look at how SuperAgers are responding to this challenge next, and then outline what you can do about it.

THE GENERATIONAL CHARACTERISTICS AND ATTITUDES OF BABY BOOMERS

Working because you have to keep working is one thing. But Baby Boomers add a second factor: they *like* working and they see no reason to stop.

Among the many criticisms leveled at Boomers, a big one is that they've always been workaholics. The Boomer attitude, according to these critics, is that working is how you validate yourself, how you keep score. According to one HR website, Baby Boomers tend to be very hardworking individuals who define themselves by their professional achievements and are driven by perks and status.

This matters because Baby Boomers account for more than three-quarters of the 65-plus population. The youngest Boomers are just under 60, but by 2030 all Boomers will be 65 or older, so their attitudes and behavioral characteristics increasingly define the entire 65-plus age group. Even if they aren't driven by financial need, if the Boomers love work, if work validates them and gives them a sense of purpose and fulfillment, then work they will.

THE REALIZATION THAT SOCIETY NEEDS MORE OLDER WORKERS

This is a relatively new phenomenon, but the topic is getting hotter and hotter as the twin effects of longevity and collapsing birth rates become more evident. Fifty years ago, there were six working-age people for one retired person; today, there are only three—and some demographers predict it will reach a 50/50 status (depending on which country we're measuring) before 2050.

The impact on public finances will also be huge: higher pension and health costs, lower tax revenues from fewer workers. It's a deadly combination that already has some governments freaking out. China, for example, is very worried about the upside-down pyramid of fewer younger people carrying more older people. The Chinese Academy of Social Sciences (CASS) predicts that pension reserves could run out by 2035 and face a shortfall of $700 billion by 2050. In a desperate effort to increase the youthful population, China has already reversed its one-child birth policy, but still faces a net depopulation going forward. CASS warns that the population could peak by 2025 and then start to decline, which would cause growth to plummet and ultimately cause insufficient demand. That, CASS says, would have a detrimental impact on their drive for consumption. That's putting it mildly. The growth rate of the entire economy would be at risk, along with China's geopolitical strategy, which depends on an annual growth rate of about 4%.

Quite apart from the scary long-term prospects, there is an immediate shortfall in the labor force, and hardly a day goes by without some new report from a think tank or research organization stating that older workers represent the solution to the problem. Can they be motivated to stay in the labor force? Can they be retrained, or their skills updated? Are there new and better techniques for managing a multigenerational workforce? (This is the first time in history that we've had four generations— Baby Boomers, Gen X, Millennials, and Gen Z—all in the workforce at the same time.) And companies are responding with new programs and policies. For example, Microsoft has introduced an "age-inclusive" program whose benefits include more comprehensive health coverage, four weeks of annual family caregiver leave, and the maintenance of benefits for employees who downshift from full-time to part-time (so at least they're not leaving altogether).

The net effect of all this is to mainstream the idea of continuing to work. Staying in the workforce past 65 will no longer be a vanity project for a relatively small number of hyperactive Baby Boomers, but an essential feature of what employment is, and a vitally necessary engine to protect economic growth rates and society's financial stability.

The future of work is . . . more work.

NEW FORMS OF WORK

It shouldn't come as a surprise that there is no single model for this new reality. Declining to retire at 65 and staying in the same job is certainly one response. But there are others as well.

Un-retirement, or returning to the workforce after you've retired, is now frequent enough to have become a Thing. As far back as 2015, a study by RAND Corporation revealed that almost 40% of workers over age 65 had previously retired and then returned to work. Some rejoined their former companies, either as part-time consultants or in a full-time job; some found new employment; some pursued one of the avenues outlined next. The point is that retirement itself need not be the permanent change in status that it is in the DefaultAging model. SuperAgers are free to change their minds, and the way they spend their time.

The gig economy offers SuperAgers the advantage of being retired from a full-time job while continuing to make money on a project basis. What's more, their age and experience (and its higher price tag that may be a disadvantage when seeking a new full-time position) becomes a competitive advantage in a gig situation. Companies can leverage all that knowledge and wisdom in a concentrated, limited-time and limited-money structure, avoiding a more cumbersome longer-term commitment. A 2020 report by staffing platform Wonolo said that about 30% of Baby Boomers were doing as many as three gigs a week.

Franchises or home-based businesses appeal to SuperAgers' entrepreneurial attitude, and buying or starting a business is an attractive financial solution. Franchises are an especially great option as many start-up elements have already been solved. According to a 2022 survey by BizBuySell, an online business-sale marketplace, 30% of buyers are Baby Boomers. In Canada, one-third of new businesses are funded by people over age 50. Another interesting factoid from Canada (per Vividata): In 2011, 101,000 people over the age of 65 had an office in their home. Ten years later, for the same age group, the number was 770,000.

Entirely new careers, also known as encore careers, are another growing trend. Some are in entrepreneurial situations, but a large number are with not-for-profits, where SuperAgers can bring the talents and experiences they've accumulated over the years and apply them to the achievement of socially important goals. In this way, Accomplishment can include more than money, as we'll see more of next.

OTHER ARENAS FOR ACCOMPLISHMENT

Let's be clear: the job front is only one arena where the post-65 life can be marked by Accomplishment.

Even the DefaultAging model, as limited and unambitious as it is, does include a few other items. You could volunteer for a good cause, but it's probably going to be close to home and you're mostly going to be told what to do by younger managers (flash that nice warm smile of yours up and down the hallways as a candy striper at the local hospital). You could continue a hobby or take up a new one—but the list is generally unadventurous: sewing, knitting, scrapbooking, woodworking. Your accomplishments will be modest, and largely limited to your own emotional satisfaction.

Grandparenting can be an important part of the mix. But again, the DefaultAging stereotype is mild and somewhat sentimental: spoiling the grandkids or serving as a babysitter (because after all, you don't have much else to do). This is not to diminish its value, of course. But grandparenting is essentially passive, or at least structured around the needs and schedules of others, and with the underlying assumption that you're not bringing much to the table.

But in the world of SuperAging, the same impetus toward Accomplishment—concrete, meaningful accomplishment—characterizes even those activities that do not earn money. Here are some big examples of what's happening in the SuperAging world. You'll have no trouble seeing how different it is from the DefaultAging model.

Volunteering means opportunity and excitement. Led by the Baby Boomers, SuperAgers are much more demanding about what they want when they volunteer. And it's been noted by the professionals who run not-for-profit organizations; many of those organizations have had workshops, or even entire conferences, on the topic. (David spoke at a large conference in Calgary, Alberta, that brought together over 30 community not-for-profits, large and small, to examine the challenges of attracting and engaging Baby Boomer volunteers.)

The previous generation of volunteers typically respected the authority and structure of the organization they were working for and didn't make waves. They were happy to earn a seat on a committee. DefaultAgers all the way. The new breed is different; led by the Boomers, the SuperAgers are bringing the same drive, the same goal-oriented approach, that they brought to their working careers. Volunteering becomes just an extension of their career-driven lifestyle.

As a result, they're ambitious. They want a bigger say and a bigger role, and they need to feel they're contributing and effecting positive change, not just putting in time. For the SuperAger, volunteering isn't just something to do to get you out of the house; it has to have an important mission.

This explains the popularity, for example, of "voluntourism"— combining the desire to do good with the love of travel. Why content yourself with selling magazines in the hospital's gift shop when you can help build a school in a jungle? Especially when it's so easy to get involved. Numerous organizations now offer online directories of overseas volunteering opportunities that are especially tailored for older people in faraway locations ranging from Ecuador to Nepal to Cambodia.

SuperAgers demand the same benefits in local opportunities, and many not-for-profit organizations are redesigning their volunteer programs to make them more appealing to this vast audience. They realize these programs need to morph from task-oriented (show up for a few hours every week and carry out tasks that are, even if valuable, relatively mundane) to goal-oriented (your work makes a real difference to the organization, and even includes effecting positive changes in strategy and outcomes). If SuperAgers are going to get involved, they're *really* going to get involved!

Back to school. Every year when it's graduation time, there's guaranteed to be a newspaper story or TV news clip about a "senior citizen" earning a university degree in their 80s, 90s, or even older. These are much more than individual human-interest stories; they're examples of a far bigger trend. SuperAgers are going back to school to earn degrees. They're sitting in the same classrooms as Millennials and Gen Z students and earning the same credentials.

The impetus here is obvious: a degree is, in and of itself, a mark of Accomplishment. And the process of earning that degree is not only interesting and challenging but has the added benefit of promoting health, particularly brain health.

There are also strong motivations on the part of the universities and colleges. SuperAgers represent an enormous market at a time when enrollments of the traditional youthful student base are flat or declining. So strong is the opportunity, in fact, that many universities are spinning off separate programs specifically targeted at the older market. Many of the programs don't grant degrees but do offer formalized courses with detailed curricula, so it isn't just dabbling, it's real learning. Two good examples are the Osher Lifelong Learning Institute at the University of Washington in Seattle, and the Chang School of Continuing Education at Ryerson University in Toronto.

Osher offers about 20 courses on a variety of topics, led by university faculty or experts recruited from the community. Chang, which offers continuing education to all age groups, has spun off a separate program for the 50-plus age group, with aims of helping cultivate purpose and enrichment, increase social networking, and "redefine later life living." There are now over 300 programs serving more than 3,000 students a year.

Learning new skills promotes longevity, and the classroom isn't the only venue. With the internet has come an explosion in online learning, with products ranging from a single how-to video on YouTube to elaborate, multi-lecture presentations, in some combination of video, podcast, downloadable lesson plan, and even an app.

There is a big uptake among SuperAgers because these formats allow for more convenience and flexibility and still deliver a disciplined and properly sequenced program of learning. It's an ideal way to learn new skills.

Here's one example. In the previous chapter, we mentioned

Sir Muir Gray, who has some revolutionary ideas about a new model for healthcare delivery, where the patient has much more to contribute and even control. He has now codified those ideas into an online training course that includes both lectures and a downloadable study guide. (There's a link in the Resources section at SuperAging.info.)

Another good example: in that same chapter, we talked to Dr. Allison Sekuler about brain health and discussed how learning a new language supports it. There are now literally hundreds of online courses and apps that can teach you a new language. The quality is uneven, of course, and you have to do a little research to find the best ones; we have some recommendations in the Resources section on SuperAging.info.

The important point here is that many SuperAgers are treating learning as a serious undertaking, and not just a mildly interesting or transitory pastime. And they have a dazzling range of resources to help them.

MAKE ACCOMPLISHMENT PART OF YOUR SUPERAGING PROGRAM

Faced with so many new opportunities and resources, how do you go about building your own Accomplishment plan?

Of course, a lot depends on you, where you are in life right now, where you see yourself in the future. Your definition of Accomplishment will be your own; it's not for us to dictate what the details must be or how far you need to go. There is no external benchmark, no universal SuperAger scale of Accomplishment, that everyone is expected to live up to. The only common denominator is a sense of both *purpose* and *engagement*, as distinct from the DefaultAging model of withdrawal and lack of aspiration.

We recommend keeping it simple, especially at the start, and then letting the action steps grow as you work your way through. Here are the three steps to get you started:

1. Define a goal or purpose.
2. Research the categories of possibility.
3. Consider a coach.

DEFINE A GOAL OR PURPOSE

When it comes to Accomplishment, the starting point must be a positive, enthusiastic, and uncompromising Attitude that you

- do have things you want to accomplish;
- do believe you have enough time (years left to live) and resources to accomplish them; and
- can therefore succeed.

It is almost impossible to overstate the importance of laying out a purpose and specific goals for Accomplishment. In the chapter on Attitude, we reviewed some of the scientific proof that people with a sense of purpose (and the optimism that they can/will achieve that purpose) actually live longer than people without that sense of purpose. The Blue Zone centenarians are a good example.

We're not talking here about a vague "feel-good" mood. We're talking about specifics: *put it in writing*. What do you want to accomplish over the next year? The next five years? Ten? Twenty?

The list will change, of course. You'll check off certain things you've actually done—the classic bucket list approach. There will be some false trails where you'll start certain projects and then decide to drop them and move on. Your initial written plan should not be seen as limiting you or fencing you in; the whole point is that it be dynamic. Essentially, we want you to be as attentive, methodical, and responsive to new situations or opportunities as you were in the management of your career. Think about the variables that you handled: you went after promotions and didn't get them, you went after promotions and got them and then were or were not happy (and adjusted accordingly), you switched jobs, you added new training or refocused your skills, you integrated it all with a financial plan, you kept tweaking and adapting . . . In sum, you were an **active manager** of your future.

We want you to bring exactly the same mindset to the management of the future you have in store right now.

RESEARCH THE CATEGORIES OF POSSIBILITY

The next important step is to make sure you are fully aware of the possibilities and resources that are out there. You may certainly concentrate your Accomplishment goals based on your personal preferences; you should not, however, limit them because you don't know what's possible and available.

We recommend organizing into three logical categories and assembling the information using the techniques we outlined in the Awareness chapter. Each category in turn sets up logical subcategories and offers a rich and ambitious menu of choices.

- Employment—paid
    - Continue with current job full-time
    - Continue with current job part-time
    - New full-time job
    - New part-time job or gig
    - Buy or open a new business

- Employment—unpaid
  - Volunteer for local organization
  - Pursue overseas volunteer opportunity
  - Pursue mentorship opportunity
- Education and self-improvement
  - For-credit courses leading to credentials (e.g., degree, diploma)
  - Not-for-credit courses at universities and colleges
  - Online learning
  - Personal coach, trainer, teacher of new skills
- Housing and independent living
- Relationships and social network

The last two points are important—so important that they each deserve (and get) an *A* of their own. Autonomy and Attachment will be covered in more detail in the coming chapters.

The rest of the list has to do with what we conventionally think of as "occupation." For DefaultAgers, as we have seen, the choices were limited, the range of expectations was small, and—very important—the supportive resources were very few. In the SuperAging world, however, there is an enormous range of information and services that can help you. And we're not just talking about Google searches. To take just a small sampling, and using only the United States as our example:

- AARP, the largest organization for seniors, has a job board and runs physical and online job fairs. AARP's Back to Work 50+ program also offers training, coaching, and job-seeking tools.
- Most state governments offer employment services for older workers. A good example is California's Employment Development Department, which

works with local agencies and organizations to
provide training to help older workers return to the
workforce or transition into new careers.

- Many private employment agencies, like
ManpowerGroup and Kelly Services, have spun off
special job placement categories for seniors, matching
job candidates with employers for both full-time and
part-time positions.

- There are numerous websites, like RetirementJobs
.com, offering tips as well as job listings.

The same range and depth of information is now available
when it comes to volunteering or other unpaid work. You'll know
best which local organizations interest you and how to reach
them, but there are also tools that can help you explore a wider
horizon. For example, AmeriCorps Seniors, a project of the US
government, matches over 200,000 people a year with volunteer
opportunities from partner organizations. Their website includes
a pathfinder tool that enables you to search for opportunities by
geographical location. There are also numerous websites that list
overseas volunteering options.

As for education, there are many websites that list multiple
programs and sources of financial support. No matter what
you're looking for, you will find an institution and a program to
suit your needs and wants.

A special note on mentoring. This is becoming increasingly
popular, as it provides you with the opportunity to pass
on your knowledge and skills to younger people. Plus, the
intergenerational dynamics can be very rewarding. But there
are hardheaded business reasons why mentorship is growing:
entrepreneurs of all ages value the real-life knowledge of experts
who have accumulated years of experience.

Many universities and colleges are employing seniors as

teachers (particularly in not-for-credit courses that are less rigid about academic credentials and tenure) or as informal mentors in study groups. Some schools actively recruit retired executives to consult on curriculum development or to offer practical advice to undergraduates so that they gain more than just theoretical knowledge. The accounting profession in the United States, for example, has formalized this as an Executive-in-Residence program at a number of universities. It's an ideal way for retirees to stay involved in their profession and contribute to the next generation.

There are numerous online resources for all these topics. We've compiled a strong list to get you started, and you'll find it in the Resources section at SuperAging.info.

CONSIDER A COACH

Okay, we have physical fitness trainers and coaches for individual sports. Or, if you want to expand the category, there are nutritionists and investment advisers. We're all familiar with many different types of experts who are available.

But a retirement coach? A trainer for reinvention?

These roles not only exist but are part of a rapidly growing field. In fact, we predict that consulting with a retirement or reinvention coach will become as routine as seeing an expert on health and wellness or exercise or investments. But who are these coaches and how can they help?

The profession is an expansion of the numerous "leadership training" consultants and systems that have been common in the business world for decades. There are several organizations that prepare trainers and offer certificates or credentials to recognize the knowledge and skills that have been acquired. The Co-Active Training Institute, for example, bills itself as "a worldwide leader in professional coach training." Formerly the Coaches Training Institute, it claims to have trained over 65,000 coaches, "including employees in more than a third of the *Fortune* 100 companies." The Canada Coach Academy offers certification as a life and wellness coach, performance coach, and total professional and business coach. It's affiliated with the International Coaching Federation (ICF), which boasts over 40,000 members in 147 countries. Most of the training is done through online courses that enable the prospective coach to progress at their own pace.

What's impressive here is the growth rate. In 2000, ICF had only 3,240 members, so it's grown more than tenfold in the past 20 years—that certainly speaks to an increase in demand for these services. There are so many more people now who are taking a deliberate, conscious look at their post-65 opportunities and seeking some mixture of assistance and inspiration.

To find out more about what coaches bring to the table and how they view the SuperAging revolution, we interviewed two successful coaches: Lisa da Rocha in Toronto, Canada, and John Windsor in Boulder, Colorado. Both entered coaching after highly successful careers elsewhere, and both have experience that speaks directly to the themes we're exploring in this book.

Next, you'll find a quiz from each of them that can help you consider where you are with life and career goals. The specific advice they offer on "what to do with the rest of your life" will vary based on the specifics of the individual clients—their age, their position (employed / near retirement / retired), their interests and goals. Covering the huge range of variables obviously lies outside the scope of this book. But both also offer some very interesting tools for self-analysis and assessment, and we think you'll find these extremely valuable, no matter what your individual circumstances may be. Both Da Rocha and Windsor also supplied us with a list of books they recommend, and we've included those in the Resources section at SuperAging.info.

THE GREAT REASSESSMENT QUIZ BY LISA DA ROCHA

Da Rocha's quiz, along with her experience and insights, offers two significant lessons for SuperAgers. On the one hand, it's important to understand where you're coming from, what attitudes, likes, needs, and desires you are bringing to the situation.

On the other hand, even as you're (quite rightly) accumulating information about what the next stages might entail, and where the best opportunities might lie, it's important not to overthink things, especially at the outset. Don't let your information-gathering and analysis go too far, too quickly and block you from testing and experimentation. Take the following quiz, checking which option you align with most.

1. My life and career have purpose and meaning that is important to me.
   Strongly disagree_____ Disagree_____ Agree_____
   Strongly agree_____

2. I feel that my talents are well utilized and appreciated.
   Strongly disagree_____ Disagree_____ Agree_____
   Strongly agree_____

3. I've defined what a "life well lived" looks like for me and invest my time and effort in these areas.
   Strongly disagree_____ Disagree_____ Agree_____
   Strongly agree_____

4. There's something in my life, beyond myself, that I am contributing to.
   Strongly disagree_____ Disagree_____ Agree_____
   Strongly agree_____

5. I believe that with focus and energy I can create, learn, and develop anything.
Strongly disagree_____ Disagree_____ Agree_____
Strongly agree_____

6. My work and life offer me plenty of opportunities to learn and grow.
Strongly disagree_____ Disagree_____ Agree_____
Strongly agree_____

7. I have hobbies, activities, and/or people in my life that expand and stretch me.
Strongly disagree_____ Disagree_____ Agree_____
Strongly agree_____

8. I embrace the fact that I am both a work in progress and perfect as I am.
Strongly disagree_____ Disagree_____ Agree_____
Strongly agree_____

9. I get seven to nine hours of sleep every night.
Never_____ Sometimes_____ Most of the time_____
Always_____

10. I eat a healthy, nutritious, whole-food diet.
Never_____ Sometimes_____ Most of the time_____
Always_____

11. I get 30 minutes of moderate exercise every day (e.g., walking).
Never_____ Sometimes_____ Most of the time_____
Always_____

12. I use strategies that help me manage stress effectively.
Strongly disagree_____ Disagree_____ Agree_____
Strongly agree_____

13. I can balance the positive and negative aspects of any situation, circumstance, and person.
Strongly disagree_____ Disagree_____ Agree_____
Strongly agree_____

14. I can accept all my emotions without getting caught up in the story or being right.
Strongly disagree_____ Disagree_____ Agree_____
Strongly agree_____

15. I have deep, supportive, and positive relationships in my life.
Strongly disagree_____ Disagree_____ Agree_____
Strongly agree_____

16. I feel comfortable asking others for help.
Strongly disagree_____ Disagree_____ Agree_____
Strongly agree_____

17. I feel connected and supported by my coworkers.
Strongly disagree_____ Disagree_____ Agree_____
Strongly agree_____

18. I invest quality time in building deep relationships with people who are important to me.
Strongly disagree_____ Disagree_____ Agree_____
Strongly agree_____

19. I engage in activities outside of work that bring me joy.
Strongly disagree_____ Disagree_____ Agree_____
Strongly agree_____

20. I have things in my life that I am excited about.
Strongly disagree_____ Disagree_____ Agree_____
Strongly agree_____

21. I maximize my energy by honoring rest and renewal.
Strongly disagree_____ Disagree_____ Agree_____
Strongly agree_____

22. I create a life of play and laughter.
Strongly disagree_____ Disagree_____ Agree_____
Strongly agree_____

The scoring is straightforward. You'll notice that the choices run in a continuum, left to right, from negative ("Strongly disagree" / "Never") to positive ("Strongly agree" / "Always"). Score 1 point for every time you chose the first option offered (extreme left) and 2 points for the next one over, 3 points for the next, working up to 4 points for every answer that was the most positive (extreme right). The highest-possible score is 88.

The test is intended as a self-audit—there are no "right" or "wrong" answers—but Da Rocha did develop some useful descriptors of an individual's "state of play," depending on their final total. We found both the categories and the descriptions to be interesting and helpful:

Score of 70–80: CREATED LIFE. You've defined what is important to you and your actions are aligned with these things. CONGRATULATIONS! You are creating your life.

Score of 50–70: INTENTIONAL LIFE. You're making great progress and spending most of your time and effort on the things and people that are a priority for you. You are living with intention.

Score of 30–50: CONSCIOUS LIFE. You are conscious of what is working and not working and have taken some small steps in making changes. This is where a lot of people get discouraged because you've been working hard for a while, but living a life that is fulfilling and exciting still feels far off. Do not give up! You're doing the right things, and it's important to persevere.

Score of 15–30: DEFINED LIFE. You've started to think

about what is most important to you and how you want things to change. You are beginning to see where in your life you are living to please others, rather than yourself. You've been experimenting and seeing what works for you. Now is the time to fully commit and determine where you want to focus and what support you need along the way.

Score of 0–15: DEFAULT LIFE. You're in the early phases of defining what is important to you and how you might create a life and career that is aligned to your unique vision of success. Your life may feel overwhelming and frustrating at times, but concentrate on small wins and keep moving forward.

RETIREMENT READINESS QUIZ
BY JOHN WINDSOR

Lisa da Rocha's practice includes people who are looking for career changes but are not necessarily close to the "traditional" age of retirement, as well as people on the cusp of retirement or newly retired. The questions are therefore appropriate to this broader mix, but we think the insights are very appropriate in the context of this book.

John Windsor's practice, by contrast, is more skewed toward people specifically engaged with the retirement topic. So his questions cover not only attitude but "readiness"—emotional, social, financial, and more. Again, there are no "right" and "wrong" answers; the value lies in provoking your awareness of the topics and the current state of both your attitudes and your circumstances.

1. How do you feel about retirement?
    I can't wait___ I can't retire___ I feel a mix of excite-
    ment and dread___ I'm not interested in a typical
    retirement___

2. When do you intend to retire?
It's coming soon___ In the next three to five years___
I have no idea___ I'm not going to retire___ I can't___

3. What plans do you have for this new phase in your
life?
I have a long list of projects and activities I want
to tackle___ No major plans, except to sleep in and
see what tomorrow brings___ I want to keep doing
"something," whether or not it's called work___ I have
some ideas of things to do, but a plan is not fully
formed yet___

4. How's your health?
It's okay, I think___ It's great; I could live to 105___ I
have health issues___

5. How important is fitness to you?
It's not something I think about a lot___ Getting
regular walks each week works for me___ I do something almost every day___

6. How long do you think you'll live?
At least into my 90s___ I hope to get to 80 or so___ I
never think about it___

7. What will you do for fun during retirement?
I have no clue___ The possibilities are endless___ I'll
figure it out; I'm good at finding fun things to do___ I
have a few things on my list___

8. How important is having a sense of purpose in what
you do?
I just want to enjoy each day without any commit-
ments___ Sounds great, but I'm not sure what that
would be___ This is really important, and I have a
clear idea of how I want to contribute___

9. How will your identity change when you retire?
    It won't change; I am who I am___ There's going to be
    a period of transition to deal with___ This is some-
    thing I'm concerned about___ I don't know___ I have
    no idea what you're talking about___

10. What fears do you have about your retirement?
    Running out of money___ Being bored___ I have no
    fears about it___ I feel anxious about it, but I'm not
    sure why___ That something will happen that will
    affect my ability to work___

11. Do you have a spouse or significant other?
    Yes___ That's not a factor for me___ No___

12. What does this person think about your plans?
    Totally on board with whatever I decide___ Not
    enthused about what may happen___ This is an ongo-
    ing topic of discussion___ Not applicable___

13. Where will you live during this next phase of your
    life?
    I haven't thought that much about it___ I don't want
    to move___ I can't move___ I'm going to move___ I'll
    let my other plans dictate where I live___

14. How do you feel about "change" in your life?
    I'm not a fan, unless I can be in control___ I embrace
    it, even when it's hard___ It's part of life; you deal
    with it___

15. How involved will you be with family during
    retirement?
    We'll get together from time to time___ I'll see them
    as much as possible___ We're not really connected___

16. What kind of social network do you have?
    I have lots of friends, near and far___ I have a handful
    of close friends, but not all are nearby___ I don't have
    many people that I am in regular contact with___

17. How prepared are you financially for this next chap-
    ter in your life?
    Super prepared; I could last 30 years or more without
    working___ I'm partway there but can't stop working
    yet___ I don't want to stop making money or work-
    ing___ I can never retire___ I don't know___

18. Have you developed a budget or financial plan for
    your future?
    No___ Yes; I did it myself___ Yes; I worked with a
    financial planner___

19. How important is it to leave a legacy?
    It's a nice concept, but I'm not thinking about it___
    This is really important to me; I want to know that
    I mattered___ I like to be helpful; I think that's
    enough___

20. How old are you?
    Under 55___ 55–64___ 65-plus ___

Both quizzes ask about health and exercises and—this part
we found particularly significant—both ask about fun. Da Rocha
asks you to agree or disagree with the statement "I create a life
of play and laughter." Windsor asks, "What will you do for fun
during retirement?"

The wording may be casual, even throwaway, but the
underlying idea speaks to a major aspect of SuperAging that
is too easy to overlook. *SuperAging means having a good time!*
Yes, it's a revolution in the whole concept of aging and, yes, it
involves significant activities and achievements that transform

the individual life as well as society as a whole. Big, meaningful stuff, in other words. But SuperAgers also want to have a lot of fun along the way. While SuperAging definitely includes growth and achievement, these shouldn't be seen as burdens. They aren't mandatory expectations imposed from some external pressure to live up to an intense new model.

So don't underestimate the importance of just having a good time. SuperAging can and should include just being playful, exploring for fun's sake, stopping and smelling the roses. That's part of thriving too. Or in Windsor's words, "whatever lights you up."

Do you need a coach, like Da Rocha or Windsor, to help you get there? It's an individual decision, of course. But we believe the rapid growth of this category of expertise should be considered and evaluated, and that the use of coaches will become increasingly more widespread.

What's Next? Answers from Coach Lisa da Rocha

After a brilliant corporate career spent in the business world, Lisa da Rocha was looking for a new path, one that aligned her personal values and professional goals. She found coaching. Since getting certified by the International Coaching Federation, she has built up a substantial practice, working with executives from companies like Nestlé, Kraft, Royal Bank of Canada, and Adobe, as well as not-for-profits, educators, and healthcare professionals on how to transition to retirement or to a new job or direction. Either way, the types of situations she encounters, and the advice she imparts, are very relevant to our discussion here. The main issue: "You're successful—now what?"

"Now what?" is, of course, the central driver of Accomplishment. It automatically indicates something active and concrete, a new phase filled with opportunity and possibility.

But how to get at it?

Because of her background in science, Da Rocha was very interested in approaching these questions from the standpoint of how the brain works. "I wanted to bring in neuroscience principles," she told us, "in the sense of, What do we know today about how we operate as humans, and how does that inform our leadership?"

She found that the very skills that made her clients successful can, paradoxically, block a transition to the next phase. Those skills typically include strong analytical and problem-solving abilities, a very well-organized work ethic, consciousness of deadlines, and good time allocation. In sum: a strong left brain.

But there was a tendency to overanalyze, to want everything scoped out before taking action, which could mean never quite taking the plunge. "So often people just keep going over and over, what *can* I do, what *will* I like, and we could spend the next decade just whirling around in these thoughts, when what we really need to start doing is going out there and testing some things. You get paralyzed in the thought, because you're waiting for some sign that you're on the right track. But you won't get that sign unless you actually engage in the process." She quotes Marie Forleo: "Clarity comes from engagement, not thought."

Another part of the neuroscience element was to understand impostor syndrome, a recognized psychological condition in which you doubt your abilities and accomplishments to such a degree that you feel like a fraud. Da Rocha explained, "Externally, people are saying, 'Oh my gosh, look what they've achieved,' but internally, they themselves are going, 'I kind of know how I got here, but do I really live up to the hype?'"

This insecurity may cause them to close off some potential future avenues on the grounds of not deserving them, or of feeling that they represent too big a leap. On top of this insecurity, there's the natural and understandable fear of the future. "The feeling is 'Okay, if I leave what I've known for the past few decades, what happens?'" It begins with "working on the mindset to normalize the anxiety and the fear, and then to go from there, to get them engaged in the process of what comes next." Process is the key word: "We're just taking the next step . . . taking the next step . . . taking the next step."

Da Rocha experienced exactly that kind of uncertainty herself, in moving from the corporate world to the unknown. "I left corporate," she told us, "and the way I described it is, I felt naked. It really became apparent to me how much this cloak of 'corporate executive' offered me some respect and dignity externally. I was traveling to some wonderful places, meeting new people all the time, people wanting to reach out to me, people depending on me—and all of a sudden, that was all gone. That was hard for me. The cloak was off, and I had to figure out who I was and how I wanted to move forward."

As she's shown with her own story and through her client work, "What's next?" can be an expansive and empowering opportunity.

Stop Limiting Yourself: Mindset Reprogramming with Coach John Windsor

John Windsor's attitude toward work is best expressed in the title of the book he wrote about it: *F*ck Retirement*.

Like Da Rocha, Windsor had a successful career before

becoming a coach; in fact, he'd had five previous careers. He'd been an actor on Broadway, a novelist, a VP of marketing, a presentation coach and consultant, and an app developer. He told us he "fell into" coaching, where he was able to combine all his previous knowledge and experience.

The provocative book title came inadvertently out of a coaching session. He was dealing with a woman who had had a long and very successful career. They were exploring her situation and her options. "Every time she said the word 'retirement,'" he told us, "it was like watching a balloon deflate. Finally, I said to her, 'This word is getting in the way. We need to say 'Fuck retirement' and find a new way to talk about this time in your life.' And then I went, 'Oh, that would be a great title for a book!'"

It's a combative posture, for sure, but Windsor is convinced it's necessary because, in his experience, too many people are browbeaten by ageism into accepting that they should stop and go no further. He cites one client in particular, a professor and prominent scientist at a midwestern university, who knew he had limited time left in academia (mandatory retirement) but interpreted this as a possible signal to leave the stage altogether. "More than once he told me, 'Maybe I should just slow down. You know, I've had a good run, maybe I should give somebody else a chance.' And I told him, 'NOOOO! You don't have to do that!'"

Not only is ageism a barrier to keep going, Windsor believes it is *the* barrier, and that it is pervasive. "Studies show that some kids as young as three are starting to have ageist opinions," he told us. "Certainly, anybody born in the 1980s or earlier grew up with this image—when you are old, you are . . . pffft. And when they get closer to that age, or what they think is that age, they start freaking out, they start compressing."

That being the reality, he describes his job in blunt terms that amount to the perfect mantra of SuperAging. "My mission in life is to get people to stop saying, 'I'm old.' 'Old' puts you in a box. From a coach's standpoint, when you stop limiting yourself like that—wow, what's possible?"

In a sense, then, it's a matter of deprogramming. "It's as simple as giving people permission," he told us. "They don't think they can turn their back on all the programming they got since they were children." A coach comes in as an independent, third-party voice, and the effect can be powerful. "Somebody who is not their spouse or good friend is saying, 'Hey, you don't have to stop, you don't have to back off, you can find something new to do that will absolutely light you up.'"

We love the phrase "light you up" because it can cover anything and everything you're doing, and isn't limited to the structure of work versus retirement. This means Windsor isn't necessarily pushing for a continuing career or a second career as being the preferred option. "I have no qualms about somebody wanting a traditional retirement," he told us, "as long as they are not limiting themselves by a definition of what retirement is and is not."

Windsor works with his clients to paint "as rich and enticing a picture as possible" of what the future could look like. "What's possible for you? What could you do if you didn't have these limitations that society has programmed for you?"

One exercise is a five-minute brainstorming where the client writes down all the different things they could do. "This taps into all kinds of little vibrations and ideas," Windsor said. "We start to pull on all those threads and find: 'Oh, there's more here, let's pull on this one a little harder.'" The future is truly as vibrant as you decide it is.

6

AUTONOMY

Perhaps no topic better illustrates the difference between DefaultAging and SuperAging than Autonomy. The desire to live independently for as long as possible is common to both groups; of course nobody is eager to go into a nursing home. But unlike the DefaultAgers who passively accepted whatever was on offer, the SuperAgers are demanding more—much more—and have spawned a multi-hundred-billion-dollar industry to cater to their wants and needs.

There is a dizzying progression of new developments, a drastic rethinking and discarding of old models of accommodation and care, and a constant stream of new products and services (many involving technology). To achieve the SuperAging model of Autonomy, you need to know about a much wider range of information than ever before.

In this chapter, we'll help you navigate the breathtaking new landscape, considering three main components:

1. Housing. Where will you live? Will you need to make changes as you get older? What qualities and characteristics will your present or future residence need to have to support SuperAging?

In the DefaultAging world, there is usually a change in housing. The assumption is that as you grow older, perhaps are now a widow or widower, and your physical strength diminishes, you will no longer be able to maintain a house on your own. Or at least, not a big house—detached, two stories, lots of fix-up and yard work, and so on. So you sell the house and move into an apartment. Perhaps it's just a regular apartment in a building that is not necessarily tailored to seniors or retirees; perhaps it's a retirement residence with a few extra amenities and some on-site care support. You downsize, in other words. You might stay in that apartment for the rest of your life, or if you get more frail, and particularly if you suffer from dementia or Alzheimer's, you might move into a long-term care home for the final phase. This model still prevails, and its terminology—retirement home, nursing home—still defines the topic.

2. Healthcare. What kind of care and support (physical, mental, social) will you need as you try to get older without getting old? What resources are already available? What new ones are being developed?

Care is certainly a big issue in the DefaultAging model. It's assumed the DefaultAger will gradually need, at minimum, some level of physical help with what is professionally labeled as ADL (activities of daily living) and, eventually, quasi-medical or medical help as aging leads to progressively more frailty. The care is personal and physical such as a family member or a paid worker who comes into the home and renders the service. Gradually, when the need for care becomes intense enough, the DefaultAger moves into some form of institutional care.

3. Money. Apart from your approach to Accomplishment (retire / not retire, as outlined in the previous chapter), do you need to rethink investments and financial planning? What new ideas are emerging from professionals in this field?

The main issue, as we've mentioned, is that SuperAgers are outliving the 10–15 years that the DefaultAging model allows for. The model is rendered obsolete simply because (a) it is too limiting to work effectively for a post-65 life span of 20–30 years, and (b) the people now doing the aging are much more proactive than the DefaultAgers in their search for independence, and much more aggressive in their demands for better resources and services.

HOME: MORE THAN JUST A RESIDENCE

The first big change is in housing. In the DefaultAging model, housing has a very limited and utilitarian function: a roof over your head. True, you might want to modify it to make it easier for you to stay there as you get older by adding stair lifts or installing grab bars in the showers. You may get a smaller place or move out altogether to a retirement residence, or, if you're really incapacitated and have no choice, to a nursing home. But the housing itself can't do much for you and your longevity other than to be relatively manageable or not manageable.

In the SuperAging world, housing is a positive contributor to getting older without getting old. Its mission is much more than just the absence of impediments. In its location, design, and amenities, it is expected to actively foster Autonomy.

The signs are everywhere.

UPGRADES TO AN EXISTING HOME

Contrary to the DefaultAging model of automatically downsizing when you reach a certain age, SuperAgers are confounding the experts by *not* automatically trading in their big homes for smaller ones. Rather, they are staying in those homes and loading them up with lifestyle-enhancing amenities.

The trend is strong enough to have provoked a lot of backlash from the younger generations who blame the Boomers for clogging up the real estate markets. Typical was this op-ed in SaltWire, headlined: "Why Baby Boomers Are Breaking the Real Estate Market in Canada." The article claims that exorbitant housing prices in Canada's major cities are in large part caused by the tight real estate market seemingly resulting from "real-estate wealthy Boomers."

What those nasty Boomers are doing is not just clinging to their homes (they do have a huge asset value), but adding more features and in some cases putting on additions that make the homes even bigger. A 2021 presentation at the Kitchen and Bath Industry Show sponsored by the National Association of Home Builders provided some eye-opening examples of these amenities:

- A home office or workplace (tying in with our Accomplishment pillar). "A home office, or flex office, is not just nice—it's a must," said one of the speakers at the conference.
- A bonus room (often on the second floor) to provide additional space for visiting family and friends.
- Designer kitchens, with restaurant-grade ovens and refrigerators. Some of the designs are quite edgy. GE's Bold Ambition collection, promoted at the conference, was inspired by fashion icon (and

centenarian!) Iris Apfel. Forget bland—SuperAgers
want daring.

- A separate vestibule just for parcel delivery. Now
you can get your packages delivered without needing
contact.

The specifics vary widely, of course, and it's true that not all
SuperAgers are necessarily spending new dollars on significantly
upgrading their current homes. But what interests us here is the
mindset—positive and proactive. SuperAgers want to be excited
about where they live.

RETIREMENT RESIDENCES REIMAGINED

The same philosophy applies when SuperAgers do decide to
move out of their principal home and into a retirement residence.
So widespread and intensive is their demand for more amenities
(including the physical landscape) that it has provoked deep
strategic rethinking in the entire retirement residence industry.

SuperAgers will not accept the more institutional look and
feel that may have been okay for their parents. They want a more
feature-rich, even personalized, experience, and that includes
paying more attention not just to the building itself but to the
surrounding territory.

One interesting new approach for the industry is called
"inside-out." You take some of the functions and features that
were previously located inside a retirement residence, and you
relocate them to the surrounding community. For example, you
take a community dining hall and convert it to a restaurant or
coffeehouse a short distance away. Now you have a much more

dynamic facility with local clientele and not just seniors from the residence. Or you can bring the surrounding community into the facility. The ground floor at the Heights at Mount View, a residential care facility in British Columbia, includes an internet café, children's play area, and community town hall. The Village at Crystal Spring in Maryland is part of a larger master plan with retail development, family housing, a spa, and a town commons. The integration of seniors and the surrounding community improves socialization and creates a more dynamic environment.

Other examples abound. In response to SuperAger demand, the trend is to encourage activity such as nature or hiking trails and walkable neighborhoods, including shops and galleries. The residence becomes interesting, not just utilitarian. Remember the Blue Zone philosophy, in which the residence "gently nudges" you toward more moving and doing? It's being deliberately designed into retirement living today.

And it's not just a residence—it's part of a community so an active, dynamic lifestyle can continue. What's more, residents can experience entirely new things. One good example is the "agri-hood," a feature of a new project in Chickahominy Falls, Virginia. The retirement community, targeting the 55-plus market, is connected to a 10-acre working farm. Residents can work side by side with farmers to harvest fresh produce, meet together for farm-to-table dinners, and take cooking lessons.

Another growing trend is to locate retirement residences adjacent to or right on university campuses. A good example is Mirabella at ASU, a 20-story continuing care retirement community located on the campus of Arizona State University. The award-winning project has been described as an experiment that blends "senior living services with college life and amenities," including shared spaces where students and seniors can mingle.

Just being on a university campus automatically means that SuperAger residents can plug into a rich menu of university activities, including taking courses. But there's more: four dining venues, a fitness area, pool, library, auditorium, and craft studios. Some of the amenities also serve the students, like an art gallery, beauty salon, and bistro. ASU student musicians perform in the dining room and bar.

It's obvious how facilities like this fit the SuperAger philosophy: activity, engagement, and creativity foster new and positive experiences.

HEALTHCARE: GETTING SUPPORT IN SURPRISING PLACES

SuperAgers seeing the home as an active provider of autonomy-encouraging and lifestyle-enhancing amenities is not the only point of difference from previous generations. SuperAgers also see the home as an ever-more-important locus of healthcare.

THE HOSPITAL OF THE FUTURE

The home, in fact, is the hospital of the future. That's what Jeff Huber believes. He's CEO of Home Instead, a Nebraska-based home care franchise organization with over 1,200 offices worldwide. "If you think about the future of the hospital," he said in a 2020 interview, "it looks a lot like your living room."

This is because of the explosive growth of telehealth (in part powered by COVID) and in-home patient monitoring tools that track key health metrics and communicate them to physicians consistently and in real time. Many of these tools will be non-wearable, radar-based detection devices, such as shower attachments and floor mats, that combine the monitoring technology itself with AI-powered analytics to actually predict—and thereby perhaps prevent—problematic events such as falls.

There will also be more voice-enabled interactions, like Alexa Together or Google Home. There will be increased integration of cameras, sensors, and voice-activated response systems, making it significantly easier for older people (even those who are relatively more frail or in weaker health) to consult with clinicians, have their key metrics captured and analyzed, and get helpful tools—all without requiring in-person doctor visits.

This is all part of the Internet of Things, in which interconnected devices capture data that is then fed to clinicians (human or AI) for fast response to health-threatening situations. Connected thermostats can track humidity, which affects health, and wearable devices like the Apple Watch can monitor sleep patterns and help detect hypertension or apnea. Age-tech is also creating products that directly help the user and promote increased Autonomy. Examples include AI-powered avatars that make physical assessments and diagnose conditions and treatment options, autonomous care robots that perform in-home physical functions, robotic exoskeletons that carry out physical functions for the disabled, and VR systems to stimulate the brain. All this technology is either here already or very close.

The business implications of all this development are profound, and the sheer size of the market will continue to push even more innovation and development. A recent Japanese study, for example, predicted the elder care market in Japan alone would be worth over $900 billion (USD) by 2025—bigger than the automobile, finance, and consumer electronics markets combined. This is a good indicator of what's coming, because Japan has the world's highest percentage of people aged 65-plus (28%, compared to 16% in the United States).

Development will also be fueled by insurers interested in cutting costs and improving efficiency. Smart home technology is already being seen as a deterrent to hospitalization, and payers are excited to see the home become an actual participating caregiver.

THE NEW MODEL FOR LONG-TERM CARE

The very fact that SuperAging is so powerful and transformative creates, in itself, a risk that we need to be aware of: the idea that the SuperAging model and the DefaultAging model are totally separate and distinct, and that no features of either construct spill over or influence the other.

This is not true. And nowhere is that overlap influence more visible than on the topic of Autonomy. The best example is what's happening in nursing homes, or long-term care homes.

To be clear, homes for long-term care are not the same as retirement residences or adult living communities. They serve those who have serious medical issues and require constant attention and medical care. Relatively few residents are younger than 65, and almost half are 85 years old or older.

It's clear that even under the SuperAging model, a percentage of people will eventually require this level of care. No matter how good a job they've done at getting older without getting old, no matter how many more years they've been able to enjoy Autonomy in their home or in a retirement residence or community, for some there will eventually be a phase of dependence that demands the more concentrated care of a long-term care home. Does this mean they enter the world of DefaultAging after all?

This is where the trap comes in. There is a temptation to see SuperAging as so separate and distinct that it has no reference to any of the features of DefaultAging. If you're a SuperAger, you're always going to be strong and active and independent.

Dependency is obsolete. The truth is more complex, but it's also much more exciting and powerful.

SuperAging is not just promoting Autonomy or independence; it's forcing important changes in the concept of *de*pendence.

Even before COVID, the long-term care home industry had a terrible reputation. They were seen as Dickensian institutions, warehouses for people at the end of their lives, dispensing care in an impersonal and often demeaning way. Nobody wanted to end their life in a nursing home!

Then came COVID, with massive death rates in these facilities and the brutal exposure of conditions that had been there all along: inadequate staff, terrible infection prevention measures, the imposition of arbitrary (and often pointless) rules, a total lack of voice or influence by patients or their loved ones . . . a mess, crying out for urgent reform. Granted that patients were relatively physically or mentally helpless and needed professional care, did it have to be delivered so coldly and impersonally? Did the patients not have any rights at all? Why did the facilities have to be so uninviting and institutional? Why did patients, including SuperAgers who had previously been so active and dynamic, have to be rendered emotionally and psychologically impotent just because they were physically or mentally impaired?

To be fair, these questions were urgently being voiced within the industry before COVID forced the issue and made it imperative for new thinking and new models. Those models are beginning to emerge, and they all follow the SuperAging philosophy. They seek to replace the cold, top-down culture of the past. Instead, they are building a new patient-centered approach that strives for emotional fulfillment, social connectivity, sense of purpose, and more activity in a setting that is much more residential than institutional.

For example, the Eden Alternative was developed by New York geriatrician Dr. Bill Thomas. Conceived in the 1990s, it can hardly be called new, but what is new is how rapidly the philosophy is spreading and how many new forms and iterations it has inspired. It was meant to address the three big problems in long-term care homes—loneliness, hopelessness, and boredom—by creating seven domains of well-being: identity, connectedness, security, autonomy, meaning, growth, and joy. You'll note how closely these mirror some of the most important A's of SuperAging: Attachment (connectedness), Autonomy, Accomplishment (meaning and growth), Attitude (joy). The Eden Alternative insists that these goals are achievable even in the face of physical and mental decline, and even where that decline renders the person highly dependent on care. It seeks to humanize that care by offering a nurturing environment that is patient focused.

Similarly, the Butterfly model derives from the Eden Alternative and concentrates on the emotional well-being of the patient. The model has grown steadily over the past 20 years and is now in place in long-term care homes in the United States, Canada, the United Kingdom, Ireland, and Australia. A key focus is on staff building actual relationships with the patients instead of simply treating care as a series of one-off transactions. A good description of how a Butterfly home works was offered by the public health department of the Peel region (just outside Toronto), which converted their facilities. Talking about the new "person-centered" philosophy, they noted: "It means doing more than just addressing clinical needs. It means connecting emotionally, which, due to dementia's impact on logic and memory, can be a powerful way to connect with people in a meaningful way. It means making the house truly feel like a home, a place we could welcome family and friends."

The idea of honoring the personhood of even severely dependent patients and continuing to promote the possibilities of growth and connectedness expresses itself in other ways; other

Butterfly-inspired homes feature smaller units with more privacy instead of sprawling wards, gardens and other outdoor facilities to promote physical activity (even shopping), more opportunities for staff and residents to engage socially and emotionally, and a greater role for residents' families.

The Green House Project is another iteration of the same philosophy, with over 260 homes in 32 states in the United States. The homes are small (with fewer than 20 residents), self-sufficient with private rooms and bathrooms, and feature a communal living room with a fireplace and outdoor spaces that are part of the living experience. The idea is to make the residents feel they are in a family-style setting and not a medical institution. "Green" isn't just a vague adjective either: the designs include large windows and skylights to let in the sun and generous placement of indoor plants.

We've spent some time on this item because we think it's an important indicator of the power of the SuperAging philosophy: even in those situations where you'd least expect any impetus toward independence and meaning, it is still possible to find and nurture the spirit of SuperAging.

MONEY: PAYING FOR IT ALL

Let's face it: the housing component of Autonomy is the sexy part. New ways to think about where you live and what it can do for you, plus a constant stream of innovation through new models of housing and dazzling tech-driven products and services: What's not to like?

Paying for it is another matter.

A vitally important matter because financial autonomy is just as important as physical autonomy. Living longer means needing more money—period. Where's it going to come from? We've already discussed one big SuperAging answer to this question in the chapter on Accomplishment. You fund your Autonomy by continuing to work. The math, at the very least, is irresistible. But what if you *don't* keep working? That's the assumption, of course, of the DefaultAging model. You retire and then live off a combination of:

- The return on the nest egg you had accumulated
  - Dividends or interest earned
  - Additional earnings if the nest egg increases in value, for example if you sell off assets somewhere along the way (your home, stocks and bonds, etc.)
- A drawdown on the nest egg, thus depleting it gradually but producing cash to live on
- New monthly income from a private pension or government pension (or both)

In the DefaultAging world, this combination of sources needs to last you for 10–15 years. Financial planners developed guidance around how big your nest egg had to be, what the minimum annual rate of return had to be, and how much you could deplete your nest egg and not hit zero before your demise. There were also various models for estimating future expenses. While there was a range of strategic possibilities, they all shared two key features. To the extent that the nest egg contained investments (as opposed to monthly income from pensions), those investments had to be conservative. Simple logic: in a decade or so from retirement, you'll be dead. Therefore, you have almost no time to correct any losses, and you're willing to forgo exciting returns for safety.

But you *could*, if you had to, deplete the nest egg gradually and live off the cash, working your way toward zero money and zero life span (hopefully coinciding). What difference did it make if you worked your way through your entire life savings as long as it didn't happen before the end? This strategy was expressed most cold-bloodedly in the title of a 1998 bestseller by financial consultant Stephen M. Pollan: *Die Broke*. "The last check you write should be to your undertaker," he advised, "and it should bounce."

Nursing a nest egg for a decade or so, even if you cash in chunks of it along the way, can (and did) work in the DefaultAging world, but surely not if we're looking at the 30-plus-year span of SuperAging.

Not so fast—maybe. There *is* a model that envisions your retirement at 65, followed by a 30-year life span. As far back as four years before Pollan's book, financial adviser William Bengen developed the 4% rule. It says that retirees with a 30-year horizon could withdraw 4% of their portfolios in the first year of retirement, followed by inflation-adjusted withdrawals thereafter. Numerous advisers and consultants have produced planning templates and individualized plans from this basic rule of thumb. The rule assumes half the portfolio is in stocks, and a big variable is the rate of appreciation (or loss) on those stocks. The rule also assumes a fixed rate of withdrawal where the only year-over-year increase is the cost of living in general (i.e., the inflation rate) rather than specific costs (like healthcare) that may spike in later years.

But the biggest problem is in looking at the actual cash that a 4% withdrawal would produce. Most of the 4% planning models assume an initial portfolio value of $1,000,000, throwing off $40,000 a year in cash at that 4% withdrawal level. That's nice, except that the mean amount of savings of the average Baby Boomer in the United States, according to numerous studies, is about $250,000. Under the 4% rule, that would throw off $8,000 a year. Good luck living on that amount for 30 years.

Which takes us right back to not retiring at 65. But it is also provoking some fresh thinking on the financial planning side as well. Three new trends are worth noting:

1. Financial planners are getting certified as "senior specialists," thereby broadening and diversifying their field of vision.
2. New financial vehicles are being developed, specifically in response to longevity.
3. There's much more attention being paid to leveraging the one asset class that has skyrocketed during the SuperAgers' lifetime: their home.

SENIOR SPECIALISTS IN FINANCIAL PLANNING

J.P. Morgan Asset Management tells them to plan for healthy, nonsmoking clients to live to 100, and that many Americans haven't calculated "what it will take to be able to retire at their current lifestyle."

Do you need any stronger confirmation of the reality of SuperAging?

The declaration is provocative, but the follow-up is appropriately cautious: "Too few Americans have calculated what it will take to be able to retire at their current lifestyle." No panic, but you have to do the homework.

And in the service of helping clients better tackle that homework, the entire financial planning industry is reinventing itself. Some of this is substantive, and some of it is simply good packaging and marketing, but the industry recognizes that it's no longer enough to simply be a good stock picker or to have a few simple models of portfolio construction (and to make your money as a percentage of portfolio value). Financial advisers hoping to serve the SuperAging market must take a much wider look at the client's present and future needs. This includes much more detailed and sophisticated analysis and understanding of future living costs (particularly for housing and healthcare). It must also be able to integrate the investment component (which, in the DefaultAging model, was pretty much all they offered) with employment income, tax strategies, assistive government programs, and borrowing strategies—a much bigger landscape, just like SuperAging itself.

In their e-book, *The Future of Financial Planning*, eMoney, which offers services to financial advisers, sums up this new reality as the shift from "the conventional financial service model and the journey to holistic planning."

As a result of this new reality, the industry has created a slew of education and training programs, and special new certifications, to identify (or if you prefer a marketing slant on all this, to *brand*) a whole new breed of financial planner: the senior specialist.

A good example is the Society of Certified Senior Advisors, which awards a CSA (Certified Senior Advisor) designation for "professionals who are able to demonstrate their competence and knowledge of working with older adults into their professional practices." The society offers an online self-study program, Working with Older Adults, covering 26 topics that include the journey and experience of aging, best practices in communicating with older persons, financial planning for retirement, investing after age 65, and estate planning, among others.

There are many other similar programs. In Canada, for example, the Canadian Securities Institute offers a Certificate in Retirement Strategy with specific training in goal setting, wealth conversion and withdrawal, tax strategies, and other topics affecting seniors. The program is designed for professionals with experience in the financial services industry "to gain a credential to reflect their specialization in retirement strategy advisory services for their clients."

In the United Kingdom, there's the Society of Later Life Advisers (SOLLA), which issues its accreditation based on four standards: technical knowledge, offering a supportive environment including resources to "maintain their ongoing 'later life advice' learning and development," knowledge of the client market, and application of that knowledge ("understanding of the needs, capacity, and financial issues" of older clients).

LONGEVITY-FOCUSED INVESTMENT VEHICLES

The industry is responding on the product side as well. Can there be newer and more effective vehicles for generating lifetime income at a reasonably attractive rate?

This isn't the place to present detailed financial strategies or plans—you need to talk to your adviser or find one (more on that in the next section). What we're trying to do here is alert you to new trends to keep an eye on. One that caught our attention is a Longevity Pension Fund, developed by Purpose Investments in Toronto. It builds the word "longevity" right into its name and offers a vehicle that is part mutual fund and part defined-benefit pension plan.

Launched in May 2021, the fund provides lifetime income to retirees with the flexibility to redeem or invest more into the fund at any time. Purpose Investments CEO and founder Som Seif explained in the launch press release: "The financial services sector can be very good at helping people accumulate and save. But as life expectancies increase and corporate pension plans disappear, our industry has ignored the development of real solutions to support people in retirement and give them the financial security and confidence to know they will be okay." Fraser Stark, president of the Longevity Retirement Platform at Purpose Investments, added, "Longevity combines the lifetime income model of an annuity with the flexibility and ease of use of a mutual fund, so Canadians no longer need to choose between having regular distributions and financial flexibility."

Canadian readers who are interested will want to do their own research; of course, this specific platform won't necessarily suit everyone's needs. What matters, for the purposes of this chapter, is that this fund is a manifestation of the churn and innovation SuperAging are driving in the financial services industry—new thinking, strategies, and vehicles—and to encourage you to expand your own horizon about what may be possible.

THE HOME AS A SUPER-ASSET

Another fast-growing trend is the leveraging of the home as a source of future financial independence.

Earlier in this chapter, we detailed the growing importance of the home as a positive contributor to Autonomy, and we saw how SuperAgers now have a rich menu of amenities, products, and services that can be installed right where they live. But Boomers (and those older) are also hanging on to their homes because they represent a game-changing amount of potential cash to help fund the SuperAging life span.

The numbers are compelling. It's estimated that the Baby Boomer and older demographic owns more than $13 trillion worth of residential real estate in the United States, and more than $2 trillion in Canada. It's certainly true that many are taking advantage of the opportunity to sell and pocket a huge profit, but they then have to buy something else—in other words, pay a sky-high price, even for a downsized property. To be sure, some do exactly this; others opt for rental. But a substantial number are looking at the possibilities of staying right where they are and accessing the huge equity they have accumulated.

There's no mistaking the magnitude of that equity. In Canada, for example, there are 12 million people over the age of 57, and of these, 9.7 million own their own homes. That's a home ownership ratio of 79.3%. Of these homeowners, 8.9 million—or 73.4%—have no mortgage. And a quarter of them (2.2 million) own a home worth $750,000 or more. Tapping into that money while staying in the home is very much a SuperAging strategy.

One way to do it, and it's hardly new or novel, is with a home equity line of credit, which requires monthly payments. Another option is the reverse mortgage, which allows the homeowner to borrow up to a certain percentage of the home's appraised value, and not have to make payments or repay the loan until the home is sold.

Reverse mortgages have been around for over 30 years, and in the early days they were seen as highly problematic—maybe a gimmick, maybe with all kinds of harmful fine print. The perception was not helped by dubious marketing, especially in the United States. But over the years the concept has become more widely accepted, and reverse mortgages are now experiencing phenomenal growth. A good example is in Canada, where the country's largest underwriter of reverse mortgages, HomeEquity Bank, has seen the value of its portfolio grow by more than 40% in the past three years alone, now topping $5 billion. According to the company's research, 40% of Canadians over the age of 55 say they'd rather stay in their current homes than downsize. "Not only that," says Yvonne Ziomecki, chief marketing officer and EVP of HomeEquity Bank, "but 45% of older homeowners say leveraging the equity in their homes should be a core component of retirement planning."

We talked with Ziomecki to gain some further insights

into the company's growth and the state of the market today. We were also very interested in what the company has learned about its audience—learning that's reflected in its marketing and advertising programs, which we think you'll find very instructive.

In fact, these insights go beyond the topic of whether reverse mortgages are a good idea for your particular financial plan. Ziomecki and her team are at ground zero, in a way, in seeing and understanding the changing role of the home, both as a financial engine and as a lifestyle component, in the SuperAging world. Ziomecki confirmed to us that the company's growth is explosive—close to 50% in 2022—and that there are strong economic and financial reasons for that growth.

Part of it is the growing acceptance of the reverse mortgage product with the passage of time; the company has been in business for over 40 years. In Canada (and in the United Kingdom) reverse mortgages are closely regulated and have more consumer protection built in than in the United States, where the early iterations of the product involved more downside risk for the borrower. By contrast, the program is structured in Canada to eliminate the risk, for example, of losing your home if its value drops below the amount of the loan when it comes time to sell. So you'd expect some steady growth as the product becomes more familiar and more widely accepted in the marketplace.

But product familiarity is only part of the story. There are two other reasons for this enormous growth, and they both play into SuperAging and what this book is all about. First, there is the incredible appreciation in real estate value, creating a significantly bigger amount of equity that could be monetized; second, there are the SuperAgers themselves.

As to the first component, we've noted it previously, and Ziomecki confirmed its importance. She told us about a meeting she'd had with a senior financial planner at a major Canadian bank. "He said that the equity value in seniors' homes has reached such a high level that it's really become the key to a long-term financial strategy," she said. He told her they were incorporating the reverse mortgage strategy into their planning advice for those who owned their own home and had substantial equity.

There's no question that skyrocketing real estate prices have created a potential pool of cash that is increasingly meaningful (or irresistible) to people who are contemplating, as a result of SuperAging, a future of 20–30 years or longer.

But who are these borrowers? What are their attitudes and expectations, and how do those differ from the previous generation? The latter question is more important because it can be instructive even if you don't necessarily need or want a reverse mortgage.

Ziomecki agreed that it's a new breed, and very different from the potential customer pool of three or four decades ago, when the product and the company got going. "They're more hip," she said. "They're more dynamic, more adventurous. They want to do more." In a nutshell, they're SuperAgers. While many use the funds as a form of monthly cash or, in a lump sum, to pay for Autonomy-promoting renovations or other amenities, there is a wide range of other purposes, from travel to starting a business to buying a vacation property. One client bought an electric car and installed a charging station and solar panels at their summer cottage. And an increasingly large number are using the funds to help their adult children get into the housing market.

To be clear, we are not recommending reverse mortgages as a strategy for all readers. And in fact, HomeEquity Bank itself is aggressive in insisting that prospective clients talk to their accountants or other financial advisers before taking this step. What counts here is noting, again, the emergence of new players and new solutions in response to the imperatives of SuperAging. We are in a period of much more creativity and flexibility, where traditional or tried-and-true formulas are being questioned, adapted, or replaced outright, all in the service of funding Autonomy for ever-longer periods of time. As well, the people offering these products and services are much more able to demonstrate an understanding of the audience, including getting rid of (finally) the stereotype of the helpless older person. SuperAging rules in both underlying attitude and in product specifics.

Understanding the SuperAging Mindset: An Interview with Marketing Executive Yvonne Ziomecki
As career advertising professionals, we've often bemoaned the failure of marketers to fully understand both the dollar potential and the mindset of SuperAgers. That's why we were particularly interested to talk with Yvonne Ziomecki. She's fashioned a marketing communications program for HomeEquity Bank that goes beyond the statistical portrait of her target customers and creatively addresses their needs and attitudes, particularly their energy and engagement, positive outlook on life, and even their sense of humor and fun.

Ziomecki developed a series of TV commercials that present her target customers in a daringly cheeky way, deliberately addressing and challenging the conventional (DefaultAging) stereotypes. For us, this is one of the most interesting aspects of the HomeEquity Bank story: they're not afraid to address the old stereotype head-on, and to have fun with it en route to demolishing it.

In one commercial, the adult children of a couple suggest to Mom and Dad that maybe it's time for them to downsize, to sell that big house and move into a condo—the classic DefaultAging action.

"Great idea," the dad deadpans. "You guys live in a condo, don't you?"

"Yes," the daughter enthuses, "and we love it."

"Great," says the mom, still deadpan. "Why don't we move in with you?"

Suddenly, the kids explain that their condo isn't very big. The commercial ends with the older couple bursting into laughter at the thought of selling the home.

In another spot, an adult daughter is sharing a cup of tea with her mom when she hears a groan and turns to see Dad coming down the stairs, rubbing his back. She asks her mom what's wrong with Dad and is told he just has a sore back. The daughter nods sympathetically and suggests the house may be getting too hard to manage. Especially those stairs. "It wasn't the stairs," Mom deadpans. "Actually, we love the stairs." The commercial ends with a long look at the daughter's reaction, at first puzzled and then amazed as it gradually dawns on her why Mom and Dad may love the stairs . . . and what they're going upstairs to do.

"We couldn't have made commercials like these 10 or 20 years ago," Ziomecki told us. "But we think they accurately reflect our audience, especially their sense of fun. It shows that we understand them."

That understanding extends to realizing that the SuperAgers want and appreciate personalized service. HomeEquity Bank uses former world figure skating champion Kurt Browning as a spokesperson. He's 55 years old, and he radiates enthusiasm and creativity. He positions the product as more than dollars and cents—it's all tied in with lifestyle and unlocking future possibilities. He often makes personal calls to clients to see how they're doing. And in one heartwarming example, he arranged a private skating session (along with fellow former world champion Donald

Jackson) for an 80-year-old woman who had dreamed of skating with him. She had taken up skating herself at the age of 58—SuperAging personified.

MAKE AUTONOMY PART OF YOUR SUPERAGING PROGRAM

There are four important action steps you can take to ensure Autonomy is a key component in your future:

1. Make it a permanent topic *now*.
2. Conduct an Autonomy audit of your current living space.
3. Interview your existing financial adviser (or find one if you don't have one).
4. Build Awareness around age-tech and healthcare.

MAKE AUTONOMY A PERMANENT TOPIC *NOW*

In the DefaultAging model, Autonomy was something that crept up on you fairly quickly. You were living where you were living, and you didn't think much about the next phase until it was right there.

The time lapse from the realization that "this place is getting too big/difficult for me" to the research into alternatives was compressed into a relatively short period of time, usually not more than a few years at most. Certainly, it wasn't a topic 5 or 10 years out.

Often, there's a sudden scramble for resources, most notably, caregivers who can come into the home. You may have had to hire caregivers for a loved one with little or no previous knowledge of what was available or even where to find it. Perhaps you were under intense pressure to find care quickly because of an unexpected medical emergency or situation such as dementia of a parent that had not yet been dealt with. Do you want to repeat this scramble for another loved one? Or for yourself?

That's why our recommended first step is both simple and important: make Autonomy a permanent topic, and do it today.

It doesn't matter if it seems that this won't be an issue for some time. You may be in your 50s (or younger) and living independently at home, physically and mentally fit, able to deal with home maintenance, and still earning plenty of money and not thinking about retirement. But this is an important topic that you don't want to sneak up on you. We're not saying you should worry about it. We're not saying you should research with the same intensity you'll want to be applying some years down the road. All we're saying is: Make it a topic. Create a notebook, physical or digital. Keep an eye on the trends. Start to build a plan.

CONDUCT AN AUTONOMY AUDIT

Unless you have some reason to already be planning to sell your home and move, unconnected with any SuperAging issues, you should assume you will age in place and conduct a formal Autonomy audit. The audit will reveal weaknesses and the kind of action (and cost) that will be needed to improve your home's ability to support your Autonomy over the long term.

You may want to conduct this audit on your own through a simple checklist (which we offer here) or engage a professional. As with the financial planning sector, the construction/

renovation sector is actively training and certifying specialists in home renovation for aging in place. In the United States, for example, the National Association of Home Builders has created a Certified Aging-in-Place Specialist credential, which includes training in "design concepts for livable homes and aging in place." The occupational therapist profession is also interested in the topic, and its members can conduct in-home assessments and make specific modification recommendations.

Why do an audit now? This is really an extension of our first recommendation: start paying attention to the topic and the issues. Even if it's just a dry run exercise and you may be years away from taking action, it will expose you to the range of home features that you may be taking for granted. For example:

- Overall
  - Adequate lighting
  - No-step entry
  - Wider doorways
  - Lever-styled door handles (as opposed to doorknobs)
  - A ramp someday?
  - Stair lifts someday?
- Bathroom
  - Higher toilet height
  - Grab bars for toilet and bath/shower
  - Walk-in shower/tub
  - Slip-resistant floors
  - Handheld showerhead
- Kitchen
  - Sink height?
  - Hands-free faucet
  - Larger drawers
  - Pull-out pantry

- • Cabinets lower, more accessible
- • Pull-down shelves
- Bedroom
  - • Should it be on the main floor?
  - • Better lighting in the closet
  - • Bed rail
- Laundry room
  - • Location (ideally, near bedroom)
  - • Front-load appliances
  - • Appliances raised 12–15 inches
  - • Cabinets lower, more accessible
  - • Pull-down shelves

These are just a few simple basics to give you the idea of what will need to be looked at eventually. It's easy to see how they relate to possible future physical issues. Hands-free faucets if arthritis makes it harder to turn taps; ramps and stair lifts for easier mobility; wider doorways if a walker or wheelchair is involved.

If these needs are imminent, we strongly recommend a professional with specific experience (and, ideally, credentials) in serving the aging-in-place market. If you're just doing an early practice run, it's enough to start looking at your home through the lens of what Autonomy will require down the road.

INTERVIEW YOUR FINANCIAL ADVISER

Just as you should do a preliminary audit of your home, you should also do a quick check with your financial adviser—or a search of the market if you don't already have one.

You know best what your current plan is and how you're doing, so we don't recommend specific performance benchmarks. There are simply too many variables that we can't know—your age, your income, the assets you own and their current values, your current housing, your current state of health, your long-term interests . . .

Instead, we prefer to suggest a menu of questions or issues you should investigate. These can be applied equally to your current adviser or potential future advisers, and they all go beyond the core issue of performance. Performance is its own category (what specific recommendations the adviser has made or the potential adviser advocates, and have they / will they produce an acceptable return for you). That component is obvious, but let's highlight a few others that are too often overlooked.

Knowledge about SuperAging. Does the adviser understand the full extent and impact of longevity and the resulting SuperAging opportunity? Do they have any certification in this area? If not, do they keep up to date on new developments? How? Do they have a coherent philosophy of how SuperAging has changed the financial planning landscape in terms of funding (a) longevity and (b) autonomy within the context of that longevity?

Knowledge about costs, particularly healthcare and aging in place. You need more than just a few ideas (even very good ideas) on the best investments. You also need a much more detailed and sophisticated approach to estimating future costs as you get older without getting old. What's happening with healthcare today, and where is it going? What about technology that may become part of your essential budget? Is your financial adviser capable of helping you develop a much more detailed plan than simply a fixed rate of asset drawdown, as under the old 4% rule? What are their information sources, and how regularly do they update their knowledge? Do they have other resources— expert consultants, for example—that they can bring on board to provide additional knowledge and insights?

Knowledge about earning an income. Does your financial adviser understand that retirement, as we have known it, is over? Do they recognize, and integrate into your financial plan, earnings from employment (full-time, part-time) or from a new business you might create? Can they offer strategies to help you leverage the accumulated equity in your home?

Ability to be a concierge of other services. Does your financial adviser have good knowledge of other services you might need, from home renovation to in-home care to age-tech, and the ability to connect you to those services? This concierge idea is increasingly being offered as a competitive point of difference by a growing number of financial advisers. Their roster of affiliated resources could include real estate brokers, building contractors, tech experts, home care and healthcare navigation specialists, and others. You may not want a financial adviser to be the quarterback of such a network—you may prefer to keep all these separate and be your own "packager"—but you should at least know that the possibility is out there, and increasingly being marketed as such within the financial services industry.

BUILD AWARENESS AROUND AGE-TECH AND HEALTHCARE

This last one feeds back to Awareness. You need to pay particular attention to what's happening in age-tech as well as with the consumerization of healthcare, both of which we previously discussed.

These two fields are exploding, and it would be a mistake to try to play catch-up all at once when your Autonomy is suddenly challenged. It's easier, and much more effective, to keep a watching brief as you go along. We have some specific recommendations in the Resources section at SuperAging.info.

In sum, the key is to be always on the lookout for new ideas, products, and services that will promote your physical, mental, and financial Autonomy. It's the same as the need for a consistent diet or exercise program; you need an ongoing Autonomy alert. Given the ever more exciting possibilities, it's certainly worth the effort!

7

ATTACHMENT

They met and fell in love.

They dated for about a year. It was easy to spend a lot of time together since they both lived in the same apartment building. Finally, in June 2019, they decided to tie the knot.

When they went to the courthouse for a marriage license, they found out they could get married right on the spot—and so they did. When the happy newlyweds were asked how they spent most of their time together, the groom bashfully said, "Well, I probably shouldn't talk about that."

The groom, John Cook, was 100 years old.

His bride, Phyllis, was 103.

Not surprisingly, their story attracted a lot of media attention. TV coverage included shots of friends congratulating them as they rode their mobility scooters up and down the corridors of the Kingston Residence, a senior living facility in Sylvania, Ohio. They were keeping their own apartments in the building, but in other respects they sounded like a typical head-over-heels couple. Phyllis told CNN's local affiliate: "[It] may be a little far-fetched for somebody our age, but we fell in love."

On one level (the fact that they are both centenarians) this is definitely a story of SuperAging. But on another level (relationships among older people) the story would have been equally compelling in the DefaultAging world. It's about Attachment, after all, and that's something that overlaps both models.

It's always been understood that it was bad for seniors to be lonely and isolated, and that having strong attachments to family and friends contributed to better physical and mental health. In fact, the desirability of paying visits to "older folks"—particularly if they were what used to be labeled as shut-ins—was well developed long before SuperAging came along. Virtually every church and community organization still runs programs to carry out such visits.

So what's changed for SuperAgers?

There are four key points to consider:

1. **New behavioral and clinical relationship research.**
    Attachment's correlation with longevity has now
    been studied from both a behavioral and biological
    point of view. Having information about how and
    why this works can itself be a strong motivation not
    to leave this *A* unattended.

2. **A doubled relationship-loss span.** The likelihood
    of losing relationships as you age—peers or loved
    ones pass away, people retire and move—was always
    present. But with 20–30 years of SuperAging, the
    circumstances that can weaken or even eliminate
    Attachment only increase, and the duration of the
    problem is obviously greater. The need for conscious,
    deliberate strategies to promote Attachment becomes
    that much more important.

3. **Uncoupling and recoupling.** But it isn't only a mat-
    ter of what happens to you; it's also what you decide

to do. In the DefaultAging model, "old people" were more or less passive recipients, hoping they wouldn't be forgotten, but they themselves weren't really contributors to that condition. SuperAgers still want Attachment, they still have concerns about loneliness and isolation, but they are contributors, actively shaking up relationships and seeking new ones.

4. **Digital relationships.** Finally—no surprise here— there is the internet. The online world exerts an enormous impact on relationships. In the case of younger generations, an abundance of research suggests that social media can be a negative force, replacing face-to-face contact with artificial and often toxic constructs. But for SuperAgers, the internet more often promotes Attachment, as we'll see.

NEW BEHAVIORAL AND CLINICAL RELATIONSHIP RESEARCH

In the past, the harmful effects of social isolation and loneliness were recognized intuitively and to some extent anecdotally, but not really probed scientifically. But today we have an enormous amount of behavioral and clinical research into what is going on, and why.

First, the facts. Isolation and loneliness are associated with a significant increase in the risk of premature death from all causes—a risk that's as great as smoking 15 cigarettes a day or being at an unhealthy weight. There's a 50% increase in the risk of having dementia and about a 30% increase in the risk of heart disease or stroke. There are significantly higher rates of depression, poor sleep quality, and cognitive decline.

None of these outcomes is particularly surprising, but *why* does social isolation and loneliness cause such damage? One explanation is behavioral and not connected to biological or clinical causes: people who are isolated are more likely to slip into health-jeopardizing behaviors (poor diet, inactivity) and remain trapped in them because they do not have anyone encouraging and motivating them toward healthier options.

This is demonstrated in a particularly vivid way by one of the Blue Zone communities, Okinawa. We talked about the Blue Zone research in the Activity chapter, describing how a team of social scientists analyzed communities with a higher-than-average population of centenarians, looking for common denominators in attitudes and lifestyles. Having strong social networks was one of those factors, and the Okinawa example is instructive.

While Attachment networks can form organically—family, obviously, but also friends or colleagues you acquire over the years—in Okinawa they also create, consciously and deliberately, a future support network. The *moai* is a support circle of about five friends, who form in childhood and pledge to be there for each other throughout their lives.

The concept originated hundreds of years ago as a mechanism for enabling a village's financial support system by pooling resources for large projects or public works. It gradually morphed into a system of small, intimate circles of friends offering mutual support. Members of the *moai* meet, often daily, to share meals, exchange ideas, gossip, and entertain. Over 40% of Okinawans are in one or more *moai*, and some *moais* have lasted more than 90 years.

Dan Buettner, the explorer and author who originated the Blue Zones Project, reported on one *moai* member who, at 77, was the youngest member of the group. Their collective age was 450! The 77-year-old described the benefits of knowing she could rely on her friends as much as they could rely on her—not worrying if you got sick or your spouse died or you ran out of money, because someone would help. In short, that it was easier going "through life knowing there is a safety net."

The Okinawan example provides powerful evidence of the benefits of Attachment. But further research has revealed biological causes as well. A 2015 study led by Steve Cole, a professor of medicine at UCLA, looked at genes in leukocytes, the white blood cells that help fight infection and other diseases as part of the body's immune system. They found that the leukocytes of lonely subjects showed an increased presence of genes involved in inflammation and a decreased presence of genes involved in antiviral response. (Interestingly, this was true of both humans and the rhesus monkeys who were also part of the study.) Loneliness apparently triggers stress signaling, which in turn negatively affects the function of the immune system.

This phenomenon was outlined in more detail by science writer Marta Zaraska in her 2020 book, *Growing Young*. Stress, she explains, increases our output of the hormone cortisol, triggering the fight-or-flight mechanism in our cardiovascular system. This is very useful; you want this mechanism triggered in an acute episode such as an infection, where inflammation is a desirable response to fight off the bacteria. But this benign (indeed, necessary) short-term response becomes dangerous if it persists over the longer term. Excessive inflammation can undermine health and exacerbate chronic conditions.

The book notes a research study in which volunteers were infected with a cold virus. Those who were socially isolated in their lives were 45% more likely to actually get the cold. Zaraska notes that while isolation and loneliness, or the absence of Attachment, can do so much harm, the presence of connections can produce beneficial effects. One is the release of more oxytocin, which lowers cortisol and reduces pain. Research shows that hugs and even eye contact can increase the levels of oxytocin.

Attachment, then, becomes not just a desirable environmental or behavioral condition, but a biological necessity to healthier aging and longevity.

A DOUBLED RELATIONSHIP-LOSS SPAN

Whether in the DefaultAging world or the SuperAging world, the risk of losing Attachment obviously increases as you get older. What's different in the SuperAging world is the raw math: the absolute size of the at-risk population just keeps growing.

Canada offers a good case in point. In 2012, there were 4.8 million people in Canada aged 65 or older, and 1.5 million of them lived alone. This represented 30.4% of the 65-plus age group, and 40.1% of all Canadians who lived alone.

Ten years later, the 65-plus population has grown to 7.2 million—almost a 50% jump. The number who live alone is now 2.0 million, a 33% jump from just 10 years earlier, but the percentage of the 65-plus who live alone has actually dropped—to 27.2% of the 65-plus age group, which represents 36.1% of all Canadians who live alone. But in absolute terms, a healthcare system that in 2012 had to worry about 1.5 million people aged 65-plus who were living alone now has to worry about 2.0 million.

And "worry" is the right word. A healthcare system that is already stretched to the limit (Canada had a particularly disastrous experience with handling COVID, with sky-high rates of death among seniors in nursing homes) now must cope with an ever-increasing number of people who face the added health risks of social isolation and loneliness.

Other healthcare systems are starting to notice. In 2016, the United Kingdom undertook a special commission on the topic, led by Labour MP Jo Cox. Tragically, she was murdered later that year by a political extremist (unconnected to her work on the loneliness commission). But her recommendations went forward in a report the following year. The report called for national measurements and indicators that would be updated regularly; clear and defined shared responsibilities between national and local government, community organizations, and individuals; and more funding.

As a result, the government established a minister of loneliness—technically, part of the Department for Digital, Culture, Media & Sports—which launched a number of initiatives. These included the creation of a Tackling Loneliness Hub, where professionals can meet and dialogue online, and establishment of a Loneliness Engagement Fund that provides grants to organizations working directly with socially isolated seniors. There has also been a foundation established in memory of Jo Cox that provides information and resources for those working to improve the conditions of anyone who is lonely.

Now we see the same phenomenon starting to happen in healthcare policy. The leap from "church visits to elderly shut-ins" (certainly widespread in the DefaultAging model) to a minister of loneliness is dazzling, and a dramatic proof of how SuperAging is driving more attention and action to all the seven A's.

UNCOUPLING AND RECOUPLING

Compared to previous generations, SuperAgers are much more ready to actively disrupt unsatisfying relationships, even at the risk of being unattached. This has everything to do with expected longevity. As a SuperAger, you believe you have plenty of time to form new attachments if you want to.

An important note: This doesn't necessarily mean jettisoning old attachments. We're not suggesting that every SuperAger wants to say goodbye to everyone and start all over. For those who have been lucky enough to have a satisfying existing network with a spouse or partner, family, friends, and colleagues, so much the better. You have a strong foundation and can now enjoy the excitement of creating even more attachments. In fact, the majority of SuperAgers are in exactly that situation.

What's different—and what's very observable—is this: where dissatisfied DefaultAgers usually put up with their circumstances, SuperAgers won't.

The best example is the phenomenon of gray divorce (previously discussed in the Attitude chapter). It became a bit of a hot topic recently with the divorce of Bill and Melinda Gates after 27 years of marriage, and that of Jeff and MacKenzie Bezos after 25 years. Of course, cynics will say that due to the spectacular dollars in play (MacKenzie got a $38 billion settlement), both couples aren't exactly typical examples for SuperAging issues. Fair enough. But when we widen the lens to the broader population, gray divorce is an undeniable trend. The divorce rate of Americans 50 or older has more than doubled since 1990, and according to a 2021 report from the US Census Bureau, 34.9% of all Americans who were divorced in the previous year were 55 or older—more than twice the rate of any other age group.

There are several reasons, and they're all reinforced by the SuperAging model that we've been describing all along:

- **Longevity.** No surprise here. Staying in a bad marriage means putting up with it for another 20–30 years. Not a small matter. Or put it the other way around: you could have a happy second marriage that lasts three decades or longer.
- **Attitude.** SuperAgers tend to be more positive, more confident about the future. The inertia ("devil you know") and fear ("what will I do on my own") that contribute to sticking with an unhappy marriage are less likely to be such strong factors.
- **Activity and Accomplishment.** Many other aspects

of SuperAging involve growth, new experiences, and new accomplishments. If you're continuing to work past 65 and exploring new interests, it creates a mental climate where you're more willing to discard unacceptable circumstances, even if that action involves some risk.

There are also some strong generational influences at work, particularly among the Baby Boomers. Boomer women, for example, came of age during the women's liberation movement, when women were encouraged to be more independent and have careers. They are more likely to be better educated and relatively more financially secure. They are proving much less afraid of being out on their own. In fact, a 2014 study by AARP found that 66% of mid- to late-life female divorcées claimed that it was they who had initiated the split.

It's important to note that gray divorce is not necessarily always acrimonious or hostile. In fact, it's often driven by the desire for more meaning or new experiences. Obviously, some of the zest has gone out of the relationship (or why not have those new experiences together?), but at the same time, introspection about one's own life journey may be much more of a motivation than enmity for the spouse or the desire to flee an intolerable situation.

Psychologist John Duffy, writing on CNN.com in May 2021, described his professional experience: more and more couples he worked with were intentionally separating, a marked change from years in which many clients stayed married despite unhappy relationships, or gradually drifted apart. He cited one woman who saw her life in chapters, and simply wanted to write some new ones, maybe with a different partner. She felt no ill will toward her husband, and hoped he'd find happiness in his next chapter too.

This idea of "chapters" and writing new ones epitomizes, of course, the SuperAging mindset, and Duffy goes on to reinforce that. "After raising kids or seeing a spouse through a career, many married people I've worked with in middle age want to reinvent themselves," he says, and marriage is only part of it. That reinvention can be about romance, but it can also encompass work, adventures, friendship, or all of the above. SuperAging, then, is not just triggering relatively more divorces but, in many cases, a very different kind of divorce.

SuperAging is also changing the nature of Attachment itself. Just as retirement is no longer an either/or, but has spawned many hybrid versions, so Attachment is not an either/or. And some SuperAgers are trying to import aspects of Attachment into new circumstances.

Take the simple practice of visiting people in a nursing home. This is not an idea that belongs to SuperAging, of course. Visits to "patients" in hospitals and long-term care facilities have taken place for literally centuries. And the dynamic of a patient being cheered up, encouraged, and made mentally stronger by frequent visits has always been important. Surely there's no envelope here that needs pushing?

Maybe not. But consider the Rayhons case.

In 2015, Henry Rayhons was charged with sexually abusing his wife. Rayhons was 78, and a former Iowa state legislator. His wife, who suffered from Alzheimer's, was a resident of a nursing home; Rayhons himself was not a resident.

On a visit to the nursing home one day, Rayhons engaged in some form of sexual intimacy with his wife. The staff at the home filed a charge: because of her Alzheimer's condition, they argued, Rayhons's wife was cognitively unable to give consent to the sexual intimacy, and therefore Rayhons had committed rape.

The case advanced all the way to a trial in the criminal court. Rayhons was charged with a felony and faced up to 10 years' imprisonment, though he ended up being acquitted by the jury. But the case, understandably, provoked a storm of appraisal and reappraisal within the nursing home sector. What are the rights of patients? In fact, are they "patients" or adult residents who should be able to have sex if they want to? Is it up to the staff to interfere?

These questions hit the nursing home industry hard. The issues spilled over from the narrow point of contention of this particular case—did Mrs. Rayhons, given her condition, really consent to sexual intimacy with her husband?—to the wider topics of privacy, intimacy (meaning sex), and "patient" rights in the environment of a nursing home. "This case has opened the door to a conversation people really don't want to have about sexuality, old age, and dementia," said Daniel Reingold, CEO of RiverSpring Health, which runs the Hebrew Home at Riverdale in New York. The home responded by writing a sexual expression policy that confirmed "every resident's right to consensual relationships." It wasn't just a statement of intent either: the policy steps ranged from training the staff in how to deal with these situations all the way to arranging rooms to accommodate residents who are sexually active. In their view, there was no reason not to encourage consensual sexual relationships among residents.

The Rayhons case certainly plays into the SuperAging issue of Autonomy and the discussion we had in the previous chapter about how nursing homes are trying to develop more patient-centered models. But it also matters in the context of Attachment.

Here we see people extending the threshold of what Attachment means beyond the bounds that are dictated by an institutional setting. The institution says visits are fine. Some physical contact is also fine—holding hands, a hug, a chaste kiss. Attachment is therefore defined as the number of visitors and frequency of visits. But the definition cuts off there, and in this case, any effort to extend that definition is not only opposed but prosecuted.

But as the Rayhons case demonstrates, Attachment can mean more. It may even carry additional benefits for health and wellness that go beyond feeling cheerful or happy to see a welcome visitor. For example, beneficial biochemicals are released by the body during sex, including oxytocin and DHEA, a hormone that helps with cognitive function. What if nursing homes, far from grudgingly allowing some sexual activity, promoted it on the grounds of improving the patients' health?

Whether it's actively ending Attachment, as in gray divorce, or changing the definition of what Attachment can include, it's clear that SuperAgers are disrupting what this whole topic means. They're taking the definitions and boundaries of DefaultAging—loneliness and isolation are bad; connections and Attachment are good—and shaking them up to have more variations, more iterations, and more power to promote health and longevity.

They also have more tools to help in that endeavor.

DIGITAL RELATIONSHIPS

The most dramatic example of how and why Attachment is different in the SuperAging world is the advent of the internet and the explosive growth of digital technology. This has the potential to overcome barriers of physical isolation and distance and to connect individuals to activities and new friends—both human and even robot. This is not, of course, to discount the value of physical Attachment, as it's certainly better to be in direct contact with people. But digital technology offers an unprecedented new win-win, providing Attachment for those who are, unfortunately, physically isolated and adding more variety to the lives of those who are fortunate to have strong networks. Both groups benefit from what the digital world can bring.

"Technology" is a bit of a misnomer as there are really many technologies at play here. These include mobile communications, the internet, mobility tools, digital entertainment, and social networking sites. A 2016 study by the government of British Columbia identified eight different technologies that could alleviate social isolation:

1. General information and communications technologies
2. Video games
3. Robotics
4. Personal reminder information and social management systems
5. Peer support chat rooms
6. Social network sites
7. Telehealth
8. 3D virtual environments

Before getting into some of the more fascinating applications, the foundational benefit is that digital communications empower people to overcome barriers of distance and stay connected. This was most dramatically illustrated during the COVID pandemic, when the Skype, FaceTime, or Zoom call became a staple for enabling families who were far apart or in quarantine to connect.

But in the case that there are no family or friends to connect with, the internet presents many opportunities to create digital attachments, and as we'll see, SuperAgers have enthusiastically embraced them. Whether it's social media in general or interactivity focused on more specific topics, the so-called older market is increasingly online and increasingly comfortable with the use of digital communications.

We already noted one good example in the Activity chapter in the context of the consumerization of healthcare: PatientsLikeMe has built an online community of more than 850,000 people dealing with over 2,800 health conditions. In addition to being a marker of how people are taking charge of their own healthcare, it shows how the damage to healthcare outcomes from being isolated can be mitigated digitally as users learn more and receive emotional support.

Aside from the immediate benefits of more connectivity and a wider range of activities, some studies have shown that older individuals who use the internet more have higher perceptions of self-efficacy and lower levels of cognitive decline.

Digital game-playing has been particularly impactful. The 2016 British Columbia study reported on a number of research projects demonstrating the myriad benefits of these games for aging individuals. Apart from the cognitive improvements associated with digital gameplay, games create opportunities for social interaction, providing "a venue for developing social capital that strengthens strong social ties, both online and offline." Games are a way to connect for those who are isolated or lonely.

In addition to what individuals can seek and find on their own, there is also a host of digital products and services specifically designed to help the people most at risk for issues of isolation and loneliness. Healthcare providers in particular are well aware of the potential here. A good example is an online subscription service now being tested by Baycrest Health Sciences in Toronto. We've mentioned Baycrest previously in the chapter on Activity in the context of brain health; they're a global leader on both the research side and the residential side of senior care.

The program, Baycrest@Home, is entirely digital and provides a suite of services covering education, activities, guidance, and therapy "for older adults living with cognitive impairment and the families that help care for them." The program is specifically designed to provide "a sense of belonging and community."

With courses (art, music, fitness), interactive groups (reading club, storytelling, travel), games (bingo, brain games), and personalized counseling, the Baycrest program is a good example of what can be delivered digitally. There are many other programs like this, and we can expect to see a continuation of creativity as an ever-richer menu of services is developed. Some programs include providing seniors with computers or tablets, and then training them to help ensure that they can and will go online to avail themselves of digital services. South Carolina's Department on Aging ran a pilot program in 2021, Palmetto Care Connections, to teach "digital literacy" to seniors, and there are numerous other examples around the world, like the Digital Literacy Programme for Seniors operated by the government of New Zealand. In the SuperAging world, everyone's on the digital bandwagon.

This is an important point. There's no arguing with the value of training seniors—particularly those in their 80s and 90s who are less likely to have computer skills and more likely to be isolated and lonely. But it must also be emphasized that huge numbers of older people do already have those skills and are absolutely taking advantage of what digital technology can offer.

Baby Boomers in particular have always been tech-savvy, embracing every new tech possibility (from the Commodore 64 to Facebook) as it came along. It's a complete myth to characterize them as not being capable of using and leveraging digital technology, including taking full advantage of its ability to contribute to greater Attachment.

For proof, we used Canada as an example and turned once again to our favorite database, Vividata, for a deep drill-down into the digital state of play. As a baseline, in 2022 there were 7.2

million Canadians at or over the age of 65, representing 22% of all Canadian adults. Here are the highlights:

- 4.5 million (65.1%) use social media every day.
- 3.9 million (about 53%) use social media to keep in contact with family.
- 3.6 million (over half) visited a social media website (Twitter, Facebook, Pinterest, Instagram) on their computer in the past 30 days.
- Over 3.5 million (about half) have participated in online games in the past month.
- About 300,000 have visited an online dating site in the past month.

You'll note here that we have included only those statistics that relate to social connections and relationships, though there are many other stats showing high rates of activity among seniors for online research, shopping, banking, and other services. This is an enormous (and influential) population, and they will not be left behind when it comes to digital technology. The positive impact of that technology on issues relating to Attachment will, in the SuperAging world, continue to grow.

MAKE ATTACHMENT PART OF YOUR SUPERAGING PROGRAM

The connections you already have—how many or how strong or vulnerable they are—lie outside our scope here. Only you know what you need to do to improve or discard those connections. So instead, we'll focus on three items:

1. Leveraging the *A* for Activity to strengthen Attachment
2. Using digital technology
3. Applying the Attachment lens to your plan for Autonomy

In all cases, our advice boils down to increasing your Awareness of what's out there. Once you know, you can trust yourself to experiment, select, and adopt what works best.

On the Activity front, we already covered a few areas where connections and relationships are, in and of themselves, an important component of a given activity. We saw, for example, how team sports might confer even stronger health and fitness benefits than individual sports. Without necessarily abandoning your individual exercise program, are there other sports you could pursue that bring social connections with them? Golf has foursomes, but what about something more unexpected? The Resources section at SuperAging.info has links to sports leagues looking for more players.

We also saw how volunteering contributes to social connection and Attachment. If you're physically volunteering somewhere, you are dealing with other people. But does this necessarily lead to satisfying relationships? As we saw, SuperAgers are getting more interested in unconventional volunteering opportunities, especially those that include leadership roles and may also involve travel to intriguing destinations. You'll meet like-minded people who want the same thing, and this could be a foundation for future Attachment.

If you think your digital skills aren't up to par, check the Resources section at SuperAging.info for some recommended instructional programs. If you're comfortable online, we have three further recommendations:

1. **Subscribe to curated health information.** At the simplest level, receiving a daily or weekly health topic in your inbox can be a valuable form of connection, plugging you in to what's going on.
2. **Join an online group.** Get involved with an interactive discussion group that may be devoted to a medical issue you're concerned about.
3. **Sign up for a class.** Consciously and deliberately explore something unfamiliar with others. Take a course. Attend a virtual or physical conference. Study a new language or learn a new skill. In all cases, you'll meet other people who are interested in the same thing—and doing it digitally can lower the cost and increase the flexibility and convenience.

Finally, there is the relationship between Attachment and Autonomy. We strongly recommend that your Autonomy audit include a look at Attachment. Obviously, this becomes particularly important if Autonomy means moving to a new location. We saw how the retirement community industry is rethinking its product offerings to include more social interaction and connection. You should, at minimum, be aware of these trends and on the lookout for amenities that promote greater interactivity with individuals and the community. You may still wind up choosing a location that doesn't specifically address this but that offers lots of other amenities that you like. That's fine, but at least apply the Attachment filter in the search process and see what happens.

In sum, whether it's individuals making strong Attachment networks even more dynamic or social service or healthcare providers targeting those who are isolated, it's clear that in the SuperAging world, tackling the Attachment deficit is a much bigger agenda item with a much more diverse and creative range of solutions than ever before.

8

AVOIDANCE

We come now to the final *A* of SuperAging, and the only one that is expressed as a negative—Avoidance. To fully maximize the life-altering potential of SuperAging, there are some things you need to avoid.

To be clear, we're not concerned with diet no-no's, as important as they are. You're already aware of the consequences of too much sugar or processed foods, and there are many good (and very detailed) menu plans in some of the books listed in the Resources section at SuperAging.info. Besides, these health tips would have been equally applicable in the DefaultAging world.

What concerns us instead are those things that apply particularly to the new world of SuperAging—problems and issues that weren't there before and that have arisen or become more acute as SuperAging itself has arisen.

To qualify for our list, then, the problem has to be something that is relatively new or particularly damaging compared to how it may have presented itself in the DefaultAging world, and it has to be an issue you can do something about if you're warned and prepared.

As well, we want to be efficient and not having you chasing too many topics in too many directions. If you've reached the stage where SuperAging is what's next, you've already lived enough years to know that life is full of problems and often the best strategy is to roll with the punches. So this Avoidance list is limited only to big issues that can impede SuperAging if not dealt with:

1. **Ageism** in general, and in the workplace in particular.
2. **Frauds and scams** are not a brand-new topic, but with a whole new digital generation of sophistication, they are more alarming than ever.
3. **Obsolete advisers** are perhaps not obvious, but the phenomenon is real and could seriously slow you down.

It's worth noting that the problems on our Avoidance list, while potentially serious, are more than outweighed by the opportunities created by the SuperAging revolution. They can't really stand in its way. That's why we deliberately used the relatively mild word "avoidance" instead of some more drastic term. With enough knowledge and attention to the details, you *can* work around them! We'll show you how to get started.

AGEISM

There's always been a certain amount of conflict between the generations. The clash of disrespectful, rebellious youth against grumpy, doddering old folks has a rich historical and cultural tradition.

"The children now love luxury" was a typical grumble from an old man. "They have bad manners, contempt for authority; they show disrespect for elders and love chatter in place of exercise. They contradict their parents, chatter before company, gobble up dainties at the table, and tyrannize their teachers."

Another complained, "I see no hope for the future of our people if they are dependent on the frivolous youth of today."

The first quote is often attributed to Socrates, circa 400 BC.

The second to Hesiod—300 years *earlier.*

We've all seen it, and we can all roll our eyes and perhaps chuckle at the way the scene continues to unfold. The flappers of the *Great Gatsby* era became the tut-tutting mothers of the bobby-soxers who screamed and fainted at a Frank Sinatra concert, who in turn became the dismayed Eisenhower Republican moms trying to stop their own daughters from shrieking in delight as they watched Elvis Presley's gyrating hips. Those daughters, after detouring in Woodstock and hippiedom, went on to become materialistic Yuppies, only to now be on the receiving end of "OK, Boomer" and being blamed for all the evils of the world.

It's how things have always gone, but not anymore.

In the DefaultAging model, ageism is definitely there, but its intensity and effects are blunted by the fact that the "old folks" have no real power anymore and won't be around much longer. People retire at 65, just like they're supposed to, freeing up another slot on the employment escalator, so there's no serious conflict in the job market. The absolute number of people living past 75 is small, so the burden on the healthcare system, or generational competition for tax revenues to fund other programs, isn't very intense either. At least, not yet.

The negative feelings that younger generations have toward older people have more to do with characterizing them as frail and helpless rather than seeing them as serious adversaries. This same lens is applied even by those who care about older people; a patina of well-meaning condescension prevails. Seniors can't do much anymore. They have little or nothing to look forward to. But they've worked hard, and they deserve an exit scene with at least some dignity built in—it's that "there, there, dear" syndrome.

In the DefaultAging model, the laws and practices that are hostile to the 65-plus age group staying active are very few and not far-reaching, since the seniors themselves view their lives as winding up. Mandatory retirement is the biggest force here, but it's rarely challenged because retirement is the norm anyway, even without "mandatory." In this model, then, both young and old play their roles, established over centuries: from the kids, some mockery during the teenage years, soon replaced by gentle condescension; from the oldsters, a relatively passive acceptance of dependence and retreat, with perhaps some "grumpy old men" cantankerousness mixed in.

But with the advent of SuperAging, this model completely blows up. In fact, it's still in the process of being blown up, and the volatility can do some serious damage.

All of a sudden (or so it seems, though it's been building for some time), the "oldsters" aren't going anywhere. As we've seen, they're becoming SuperAgers who eagerly look forward to and fully intend to optimize the next phase of their lives. They don't see themselves as helpless. They're not automatically retiring "on schedule," which means, to the underemployed or wage-stagnant younger generations, that they're clogging up the job pipeline. Neither are they selling their valuable homes in big enough numbers, so they're clogging up the real estate market as well, making housing less affordable for the next generations coming in behind. (Or so goes the accusation.)

What's more, they vote in droves—about 6 of every 10 ballots cast in the United States, Canada, and the United Kingdom are from those who are 50 years old or older—so they have the power to seriously influence public policy. The best example is the Brexit vote in 2016, when only 20% of the 18-to-24-year-old group were in favor of the United Kingdom leaving the European Union, while almost 60% of pensioners were in favor. Since it was decided in favor by only 1.3 million out of 33 million votes cast, the influence of the pensioners was decisive.

The stakes, then, are much higher now. The old folks are no longer an object of benign eye-rolling. For many, they've become the enemy—greedy seniors who made sure to take for themselves and are now leaving a big mess for the younger generations to cope with. And they *still* won't leave the stage!

Thus, "OK, Boomer."

What may have started off as just a cute phrase, laced with typical Millennial irony, quickly morphed into vicious all-out attacks. Article after article blaming the Boomers for lack of job opportunity coupled with inadequate wages, skyrocketing and unpayable student debt, expensive housing that extinguishes the dream of home ownership, and of course (as if the Boomers all got together in a hotel room and dreamed this up all by themselves) climate change.

Result: a steady stream of critical books, articles, blog posts, podcasts, and YouTube videos, all excoriating the Baby Boomers. A Google search for "greedy seniors" instantly produced 3.1 million results. A similar search on YouTube produced hundreds of videos, including several TikTok compilations that each generated over a million views. The trend shows no sign of letting up. For example, in April 2022, Jessica Townsend, one of the leaders of the radical British environmental group Extinction Rebellion, said that "rich Boomers" should be euthanized for causing climate change. Townsend is 59 and so, technically, a Boomer herself, but she noted she would be exempt because she isn't rich. Okay, then (Boomer).

Are we being unduly alarmist here? Does all this matter?

Can't we dismiss it as just another wrinkle in the old versus young attitudinal dance that has played itself out in our culture for thousands of years?

The difference this time is that ageism is no longer just a mild sociocultural attitude. It has hardened and become more active and concrete, and therefore it threatens the SuperAging mission.

- **Ageism in the workplace.** Some progress has been made, driven particularly by an emerging shortage of workers and the increasingly desperate need for companies to retain older workers and even recruit them back out of retirement. But strong resistance remains, and it's a serious impediment to SuperAgers who want to work past 65.

- **Ageism in the marketplace.** On this front, it's more a matter of ignorance and indifference than malice. Marketers have massively underestimated the scale and power of SuperAgers as consumers, which in turn has retarded the development of new and better products and services. The tide is turning (slowly, slowly), but it's up to SuperAgers to create a real push here.

- **Ageism in the political arena.** This is where campaigns such as "OK, Boomer" are unambiguously malign. There's always been a fight for the allocation of scarce government resources—childcare versus pensions, student debt relief versus healthcare. But the campaign to portray Boomers as having hogged too many resources and deserving of little or nothing further can influence public policy against the rights and interests of SuperAgers, who are emphatically not at the end of the road.

These issues matter and require a response. You can undertake individual actions on the six other *A*'s, but you also need to be doing it in an environment that supports and encourages the SuperAging revolution. Ageism is a cancer to that environment. In fact, we could probably upgrade the *A* from Avoidance to Abolition in the case of ageism. It's that serious.

AGEISM IN THE WORKPLACE

We live in an era that proclaims its devotion to ending discrimination in the workplace. Companies eagerly embrace the doctrine of diversity, equity, and inclusion (DEI). A tide is turning where HR departments enthusiastically proclaim DEI as part of their hiring criteria and run programs to take the temperature of the workplace to make the necessary adjustments, both to the makeup of the new hires and to the attitudes of existing employees. It's all good (and much needed), but it's interesting that in an overwhelming majority of situations, these efforts still do not extend to older workers. In fact, an eye-opening 2021 research study showed that those who are most opposed to discrimination on other issues, such as sexism and racism, are the very ones who are most hostile to older workers.

The study probed the attitudes of 354 subjects and was able to measure their degree of liberalism and the degree to which they displayed "egalitarian advocacy." It found that the more respondents supported and participated in programs to advance equality, the more hostile they were to sexism and racism. Okay, that follows logically. But what about ageism?

The researchers then presented the respondents with a number of statements that were openly critical of older people and asked them to express their agreement or disagreement on a scale from "strongly agree" to "strongly disagree." They also explored what they called the Succession Principle—the idea that at a certain age, people should step out of the way to give others a chance. It turned out that those who were most hostile to older people, and most ready to support the Succession Principle, were the same people who scored highest on the "egalitarian advocacy" scale with respect to other topics.

So why would the more "egalitarian" respondents be less likely to support older members of society? The researchers hypothesized that it comes down to the perception of older people as having possessed power and resources that should now be handed down. In the face of dwindling resources, they found, "egalitarian advocacy might be more likely to predict discrimination against older individuals and prioritize women and racial minorities in the process."

This is an extremely important finding because it demonstrates that ageism is not just a factor in the environment that is coincidental with SuperAging; it can be driven by SuperAging. SuperAgers are not acting the way they are supposed to based on the DefaultAging model. To the contrary, SuperAgers are staying in the game, and it is precisely for that reason that the new, more aggressive, and hostile version of ageism is manifesting itself.

This was demonstrated clearly by an AARP study in 2017 (ironically, the 50th anniversary of the passage of the Age Discrimination in Employment Act).

- 61% of respondents said they'd either seen or experienced age discrimination in their workplace.
- 38% said they thought ageism was "very common."
- Over half thought that age discrimination began when workers were in their 50s.
- 16% said they had not been hired for a job they applied for because of their age.
- 12% said their age caused them to be passed over for a promotion.

Is it getting any better? There are some encouraging signs. More companies are recognizing that they need older workers for the simple reason that there aren't enough younger ones. They're introducing upskilling (teaching employees additional skills), allowing more flexible hours, and enhancing benefits. AARP developed an Employer Pledge Program, under which companies could publicly express their support for a more age-inclusive workforce, as well as participate in online job fairs and career networking expos to recruit more older workers. More than 1,000 companies, including AIS, Microsoft, Marriott, and Macy's, signed the pledge.

But there's a long way to go. And there are things you can do to help yourself and the process of reform, which we'll review at the conclusion of this chapter.

AGEISM IN THE MARKETPLACE

At first glance, ageism in the marketplace might look like a tougher sell than ageism in the workplace. Yes, it's undoubtedly true—almost no marketers really "get" the older consumer—but is it necessarily a problem? If marketers feel like forfeiting a piece of global consumer spending power approaching $15 trillion a year, that's their problem, isn't it? How does that stop SuperAgers from happily carrying on?

It hurts in two ways, which we'll get to. But first let's take a quick look at just how bad the disconnect is. It's stark and simple: the overwhelming majority of marketers and their ad agencies are still stuck firmly in the DefaultAging world. In this scenario, the "older" consumers are:

- Increasingly weak, confused, passive
- Not big spenders (fixed incomes)
- Not new-product explorers (their brand preferences

are already fixed in place, so why bother chasing them?)
- Not good candidates for longer-term brand awareness and development (because they'll soon be dead)

Why are advertisers and their agencies so clueless? A good answer is offered by Martha Boudreau, chief communications and marketing officer of AARP, in a 2021 interview in Forbes: "The average age of a creative director in advertising is 28 years old, so their perspective on the 50-plus consumer lifestyle has not been forged by experience," she says. Agencies just aren't interested in pursuing the over-50 demographic. As Boudreau points out, according to a 2019 survey by Grey London, 70% of her industry colleagues had not seen a brief on this demographic in a year or more.

Not surprisingly, then, these consumers are almost completely missing from advertising today. To take just one category: the majority of automobiles are purchased by people over the age of 50. But when was the last time you saw a person of this age in a car commercial?

To the extent that they do appear in commercials (excluding more obvious "senior" categories like prescription drugs, stair lifts, or incontinence products), older people are often portrayed with considerable humor as being helpless and befuddled. Women, BIPOC, and LGBTQ people have made headway in rightly insisting they be represented more accurately in advertising, and older people can too.

But the older consumer is still not there. In 2019, AARP reported on an analysis based on a random sampling of 1,116 advertising images from popular brands. Only 13% showed older people working. Less than 5% showed older people engaged with technology even though close to 70% of people aged 55–73 own a smartphone.

It should come as no surprise that older consumers notice. According to a 2021 AARP survey, 62% of consumers over the age of 50 agreed with the statement: "I wish ads had more realistic images of people my age." And 47% agreed that "ads of people my age reinforce outdated stereotypes."

And this lack of representation hurts SuperAgers in two specific ways:

1. It hides the SuperAging revolution, which in turn spills over into more ageism in the workplace and the political arena (which we'll explore next).

While advertising has always had credibility issues when it comes to believing or not believing the claims of a specific brand or product, it does have a massive influence on portraying society as a whole and in setting up models and memes that people believe in. Advertising is working hard (if not intentionally or maliciously) to perpetuate DefaultAging as the defining condition of aging. In the ad world, getting older without getting old is a contradiction; getting old *means* getting old. This reinforces, among other things, the Succession Principle—if older people are truly "done," it becomes much easier to justify the argument that they should just shut up and get out of the way. Ageism in marketing punishes more than just the marketers who fail to sell products to a large and growing audience; it contributes directly to a cultural climate that is directly hostile to the SuperAging agenda. All SuperAgers should fight against this.

2. It slows down the pace of developing new products and services, or inadequately communicates valuable ones, leading to less uptake.

In some categories, like medical research, companies understand the SuperAging phenomenon very well and are pouring billions of dollars into accelerating it even further. But in others, the lack of marketing awareness around who the older demographic is, what they know and think, and how they behave can put a serious dent in the sales of products. This happens even in categories with products and services specifically aimed at older people and is detrimental to both the company and the very people the products are designed to help.

A good example is health and fitness apps. In 2022, the HealthDay/Harris Poll found that an alarmingly high number of seniors with chronic health problems (like heart disease or diabetes) are not using apps that could help them. In fact, only 14% said they were using an app specifically tailored to helping them manage their condition. Why not? Because they felt they didn't need to constantly track their health, and because they had worries about privacy and security.

Both these negatives could have been overcome with better communication from the producers of the apps. Harris Poll vice president Kathy Steinberg was quoted in an article that reported on the research: "There's certainly room for the providers of these apps and developers of these apps to help educate consumers."

The problem extends to bigger and more extensive technology, particularly so-called age-tech designed to promote aging in place. We covered some of these developments in the chapter on Autonomy. The tech is fine, but the marketing lags. Laurie Orlov, who runs the most authoritative blog covering this industry, points out that "training services tend to lag the pace of tech change." This isn't necessarily due to false assumptions about the audience, but it does involve failure to dig deeper and understand the real needs of whom you're selling to. After all, if you've designed the product with those people in mind, how can you not then understand their specific communication needs? You'd think it would be obvious. But it isn't quite there yet. The result is not only lost sales for the marketers but lost opportunities for the consumers to better their lives.

AGEISM IN THE POLITICAL ARENA

In any democracy, the political arena is a complex jungle of competing wants and needs that are put forward (whether badly or effectively) by various interest groups—unions, corporations, trade associations, think tanks, single-issue causes, identity groups, taxpayer groups, and more. All want more government programs to favor their needs and interests, and all want a bigger piece of the government spending pie.

It's always been this way.

It's always been true, as well, that the clamor sometimes includes attacks on rival interests. But in the past, these attacks were careful, focusing on rivals who could readily be painted (and thus demonized) as powerful and well organized. Good examples—and here, we're speaking of the imagery only—were greedy corporations like banks, corrupt union bosses, and overpaid civil servants.

What did not happen in the past were attacks on ordinary people, even those from different demographic groups who might be competing for government largesse. Groups might push for their own agendas, but they left other groups alone. This was certainly true of seniors, who, as we have seen, might be the subject of pity and paternalism, but were not vilified as rivals for the rewards. How could they be? The very premise of that pity and paternalism rested on their helplessness—the dominant feature of the DefaultAging model.

True, the needs of seniors might be ignored or underfunded, but the seniors themselves were not seen as a nefarious group that needed attacking. They had no power. They were dependent on the goodies that society chose to dole out, and to the extent that they had a voice (even a relatively powerful voice like AARP), it was one of gentle prodding mixed with gratitude. Like Oliver Twist, they took their bowls up to the public trough and said please and thank you. It was difficult, if not impossible, to portray them as a threat. Besides, their lives were soon going to be over anyway.

But the advent of SuperAging has changed all that. Not surprisingly, ageism spills over into the general culture and, ultimately, the political arena. Commentators seem free to recommend drastic action to strip older people of their benefits and their political power. The hostility is vivid and often hysterical. Here is just a small sampling:

- As far back as 2009, the idea that aging equaled "generational theft" was being put forward. An opinion piece on the ABC News website had the headline: "Are the elderly committing generational theft?" Author John Stossel argued, as the subhead confirmed, that it was "time for America to do less for its senior citizens." He was sixty-two when he wrote this. Some may wonder if he was willing to be first in line to have less done for himself.
- In 2010, David Willetts, then a British MP (now a member of the House of Lords), wrote a book called *The Pinch*, in which he argued that British Baby Boomers "took their children's future," thanks to real estate appreciation and generous state pensions. He advocated a government grant of £10,000 to every young person when they turned 30.
- A February 2020 op-ed in the *New York Post* was headlined: "Gen X-ers are being stifled by greedy Boomers who refuse to retire." Author Matthew Hennessey wrote, "Once upon a time, they wouldn't trust anyone over 30. Now they won't let anyone under 60 near the corner office—or the Oval Office." And this is not framed as a Good Thing—Boomers,

he suggests, have made American institutions fundamentally worse on the whole.

- A 2013 op-ed in *Philadelphia* magazine offered five reasons the Baby Boomers were the worst generation, noting in the subhead: "Ten thousand are retiring every day. Good riddance." The Boomers' list of sins, according to author Gene Marks (who was born one year too late to be a Boomer himself), included creating an unsustainable national debt; lavish safety nets for themselves; the unaffordability of healthcare (because it needs to pay for unhealthy Boomers); racism, sexism, and homophobia (Boomers, he says, are actively working against women in business, gay marriage, and immigration reform); and the state of the environment.

- A search of only a few seconds on Amazon yielded these book titles:
  - *A Generation of Sociopaths: How the Baby Boomers Betrayed America*
  - *Boomers: The Men and Women Who Promised Freedom and Delivered Disaster*
  - *The Theft of a Decade: How the Baby Boomers Stole the Millennials' Economic Future*
  - *OK Boomer, Let's Talk: How My Generation Got Left Behind*

What's important here is not the specific complaints about the current state of affairs or the policies that would improve things, but the conscious and deliberate anger in the language and the dangerously simplistic attachment of blame solely to the older generation. To be fair, there are indeed challenging policy issues that are the direct result of longevity and SuperAging, and we have presented some of them in the preceding chapters.

What happens to pensions when people have 20-plus years of life remaining after age 65? How is healthcare funded in a new world of dazzling high-tech equipment and expensive breakthrough drugs? What about education? What about housing?

Political debate and policy solutions must now encompass a much wider landscape than what prevailed in the DefaultAging model, and SuperAgers are not complaining about a broader and more far-reaching dialogue. But they do have the right to push back against the current hysteria, not only because it's morally wrong but because it directly impedes the SuperAging agenda.

There are some actions that can be taken, and we'll present them in the final section of this chapter.

But first let's move on to the other two items in our Avoidance list. They differ from the ageism problem in that they're more responsive to individual action. Whereas you can't eliminate ageism as a factor in the environment in which you have to operate, you can avoid frauds and scams and obsolete advisers, reducing their negative impact on your SuperAging program to near zero.

FRAUDS AND SCAMS

Older people have always represented a fertile ground for fraudsters and scam artists in search of victims. They were more likely to be living alone with nobody close at hand to help them resist scammers or keep watch over their finances to quickly identify when damage had been done. Older people were also more likely to be unfamiliar with scamming techniques or too timid to object to a fraudster's pitch. And if they realized—too late—that the scam had worked, they were often embarrassed at their own gullibility and therefore reluctant to report the scam to the authorities. And the final kicker: due to pensions or other age-related benefits, they often had large sums of money on hand. In sum, perfect targets.

In the DefaultAging world, the techniques basically involved mail order, telephone, and door-to-door contact. Overpriced merchandise, fake brand names or forgeries, goods paid for but never delivered, magazine subscription scams . . . the list went on and on.

But with the advent of the internet, things have really kicked into high gear. Now the fraudsters can go far beyond selling bogus merchandise or collecting money and not delivering the goods. Now they can steal identities and crash into bank accounts. And the victims aren't just the stereotypical old folks of DefaultAging. Now digital technology makes it possible for the scammers to attack everyone at once, cheaply and efficiently. You can be a tech-savvy SuperAger at the top of your game—you're still going to get hit.

And this is the key: You're going to get hit. And hit again and again.

Therefore, the topic requires constant scrutiny and attention. Smart SuperAgers will want to keep up to date with what's going on because new frauds and scams are constantly being developed. They will also want to build and maintain effective defensive shields.

Even a quick, and by no means exhaustive, survey of frauds and scams now in play reveals a mind-boggling breadth of tactics and techniques. Here are some of the scarier ones in play:

- **Phishing.** The crook poses as a legitimate institution and contacts the target victim by email, phone, or text message, then fools the victim into providing sensitive information like banking or credit card details or passwords. With that information, the criminal can then access bank accounts, use credit cards, or even steal identity altogether.

- **Zoom phishing.** Scammers love to take advantage of hot trends. The Zoom version of phishing is to send an email (complete with Zoom logo) telling you that your account has been suspended. To restore it, all you have to do is click on the link provided in the email. Once you click on the link, the scammers can then install malware into your computer, and they're away to the races. According to the AARP, citing the Better Business Bureau, by the spring of 2022 there were over 2,000 fake Zoom-themed internet domains registered.

- **Fake shopping sites.** The merchandise looks genuine (it's been copied off the websites of legitimate online retailers), and the prices are very attractive. So the victim makes a purchase, entering their credit card data. Then the goods are never delivered. Or a cheap knockoff is delivered, bearing no resemblance to what was ordered. Many of these fake sites are promoted on social media, making it easier to access them and more important than ever to be vigilant.

- **Fake Medicare cards.** This could be by email or phone. The scammers claim to be from Medicare and promise enhanced benefits in return for a small payment. Or no payment—just verify your current Medicare ID number. Needless to say, there is no enhanced card, so if you paid any money, it's gone. Worse, if you've given out your Medicare ID number, you've provided another gateway into your banking and credit card information.

- **Accidental funds transfer.** The victim receives an official-looking notification from a payment service (it could look like it really comes from PayPal, for example) stating that an amount of money has accidentally been deposited in their account, and requesting it be returned. The victim complies, only to discover that the "accidental" deposit never happened in the first place.
- **Fake lottery win.** The victim receives a notification that they've won a lottery but they need to remit a small fee (usually $1,000 or less) for sales taxes or administrative services before the prize money can be sent. The victim pays the fee, then gets nothing.
- **Social Security scam.** The victim gets a phone call from a Washington, DC, number and a menacing message tells you your Social Security number was compromised and used in a crime. You'll be arrested and prosecuted if you don't send a fee to fix the situation. In some cases, they'll even refer you to a website where you can see the name and picture of the agent making the call. Both the call and the website are fake, of course, and you'll never recover any money you pay as a fee.
- **Security breach** on your IP address, email, credit card, bank account, or Amazon order. This often comes in as a text message, which gives it an added veneer of urgency and authenticity. You're told there's a big problem on your account, and you need to click on the link in the message to get it resolved. Once you click, of course, the scammers are inside your system.
- **Counterfeit drugs.** You're directed to an online

site where you can buy prescription drugs at a big
discount. The transaction goes through, but the
drugs are bogus.

• **Grandparent emergency call.** The victim gets a
phone call from a youthful-sounding voice, saying,
"Hi, Grandma" or "Hi, Grandpa," and then, "Guess
who's calling you!" The unsuspecting grandparent
blurts out the name of a grandchild. The voice then
says "Right!" and then continues on, now posing
as that grandchild, to spin a tale of an emergency
requiring the grandparent to send money right away
. . . and not to tell the parent.

This is just a tiny sampling of what's out there. In some
cases, the scam only costs the victim a few hundred dollars (the
scammers make it up in volume); in other cases, the stakes go
all the way to complete penetration and takeover of the victim's
computer and financial assets.

It's been estimated that at least 5% of seniors fall victim to
frauds and scams every year, which would place the number
of victims literally in the millions. In the United States alone,
according to FBI estimates, frauds and scams cost seniors $3
billion a year.

We'll explore some of the many preventive measures that
can be taken to avoid these frauds and scams in the concluding
section of this chapter.

OBSOLETE ADVISERS

The third item on our Avoidance list is the obsolete adviser,
usually a financial planner or a doctor who is not up to date on
SuperAging and whose advice should therefore be viewed with

great caution, if not ignored altogether. We've already touched on this topic in a previous chapter, but it's important enough to be amplified again here.

We must acknowledge that this is a tricky issue. In many cases, the adviser will be someone whom the SuperAger has known and trusted for years, if not decades, and the advice rendered is certainly not motivated by ill will. There may also be long-standing personal relationships underpinning the professional ones, and the SuperAger may find it uncomfortable, if not downright embarrassing, to suddenly be seen challenging advice that was previously accepted without question.

So we want to be very careful here, and emphasize that we are by no means issuing a blanket recommendation to ditch current advisers and find new ones. Everyone must carefully evaluate their own situation and decide on necessary steps, timing, and style of dialogue and decision-making.

The issue cuts deeper than whether the adviser is fully up to date on the entire scope of the SuperAging revolution, though it's likely they aren't. It's one thing for the adviser to not fully appreciate the revolution. It's an altogether different problem if the adviser is clinging to the obsolete DefaultAging model and basing diagnoses on that model. If that happens, the adviser can do actual harm.

The best example is with healthcare.

In the above section on ageism, we talked about the workplace, the marketplace, and the political arena. But there's another venue to worry about—the consulting room.

Consider a shocking study published in 2020 in the *Gerontologist*. Its lead author was Becca R. Levy, a professor at Yale School of Public Health. The study examined the eight most expensive health issues for people over 60 to see if there were any differences in healthcare costs between people who experienced differing levels of ageism in their treatment. The conditions studied were cardiovascular disease, chronic respiratory disease, musculoskeletal problems, diabetes, treatment of smoking, mental issues, noncommunicable diseases, and injuries.

Ageism was characterized by one or more of three things: outright age discrimination (denying treatment because the patient was seen as too old to benefit from it), using negative stereotypes about older people (being condescending, using "elderspeak" or infantilizing language), and negative perceptions that the older people themselves may have had about their own aging.

The results were mind-boggling. Ageism often produced measurably worse outcomes. It added to patient stress, thus jeopardizing cardiovascular strength. Patients with negative self-image performed worse on cognitive tests and were more likely (perhaps from a feeling of hopelessness) to forget to take their prescription drugs. The incidence of the eight health conditions under study was higher in the group that experienced the most ageism, and over 17 million cases per year of those conditions could be attributed to ageism. Based on those findings, the researchers concluded that ageism added $63 billion a year to healthcare spending in the United States.

Bottom line: If your doctor is ageist, even in the relatively benign patronizing style of the DefaultAging era, it can seriously undermine your health.

INCLUDE AVOIDANCE IN YOUR SUPERAGING PROGRAM

AVOIDING AGEISM

As a general rule, the closer ageism gets to your individual situation or specific needs and wants, the more leverage you have. Tackling the entire macro problem of ageism is unlikely to produce much more than emotional satisfaction for people who are combative and enjoy punching back. We're not saying you shouldn't send letters to the editor, post angry Tweets, or engage in face-to-face protest when you encounter ageism, we're just saying you need to be realistic about how little these actions are likely to accomplish. A more productive move would be to join organizations that already have anti-ageism campaigns and well-established communications and public policy lobbying channels. Examples would be AARP in the United States, CARP in Canada, Age UK in the United Kingdom, and COTA in Australia. These organizations all do valuable work and become more powerful the more members they have. In addition, they may offer better opportunities for individual action and involvement in the cause than you could generate on your own.

These organizations are also effective voices in the political arena. They mobilize votes and remind politicians that the "older" age group typically accounts for more than half the ballots cast in elections. They help ensure that the needs and wants of SuperAgers are reflected in public policy, and, to the extent that legislation can curb ageism in the workplace or marketplace, they fight for appropriate action.

But public policy can only go so far. Individual action is much more immediate. Let's look at what you can do on your own. We'll focus on two areas:

1. Fighting against ageism in the workplace, either with a current employer or in job-seeking
2. Fighting against ageism in the marketplace

IN THE WORKPLACE

Age discrimination in the workplace is illegal.

In the United States, the Age Discrimination in Employment Act was passed in 1967 and forbids age-based discrimination against anyone at least 40. In Canada, it's prohibited through a number of laws at the provincial level, with slight variations by province, but the overall effect is to ban ageism in the workplace. In the United Kingdom, the Equality Act of 2010 bans age discrimination unless the employer can show it is objectively justified; for example, a worker may be too old to perform a required job function. In Australia, the Age Discrimination Act of 2004 bans ageism.

SuperAgers who believe they are experiencing age discrimination in their workplace should have no hesitation in filing a complaint with the appropriate authorities. Scathing reviews on employer-rating websites like Glassdoor can also be effective. Employers are becoming much more sensitive to this issue, particularly if there is a possibility of public exposure. In extreme situations, individual and class action lawsuits should be considered. In 2019, Google was hit with a class action suit over ageism in its hiring practices and paid a settlement of $11 million to more than 200 job seekers aged 40 years or older.

Bottom line: It may make sense to try to solve this, at least initially, through internal dialogue and sweet reason. The individual SuperAger is the best judge of how intense the problem is and the likelihood of a constructive response from colleagues or from HR. But the laws are there for a reason, there are complaint and enforcement procedures, and it would be foolish not to employ them.

If a complaint is filed, employment law experts advise to be on the lookout for, and carefully document, any negative changes in attitude or behavior by the company toward the complainant. Evidently, it's easier to win a lawsuit if there's been retaliation.

The hiring front is another inherently more insidious matter because in the absence of egregious behavior by an interviewer, it can be difficult to prove that ageism is in play. If a SuperAger's résumé got no response or if an interview did not result in an offer, can it necessarily be established that the problem was due to ageism? Unless a reasonably large pool of similarly aged and qualified applicants who were rejected can be assembled (like the 200-plus plaintiffs in the Google action), the answer is likely to be no.

Therefore, the best strategy is to take action ahead of time to minimize the effect of ageism and place the résumé in a more favorable light. There are numerous résumé experts who can help with this, from offering general advice all the way to writing the actual résumé. We checked several resources, and here are a few of the key tips they offered:

- Don't include work history from more than 15 years ago. Hiring managers are more interested in your recent history, and besides, for the SuperAger the more recent history is likely to consist of very senior positions.
- Forget talking about your objectives or why you want the job and focus on your qualifications. The trend today is to have a professional summary, usually one paragraph, highlighting your accomplishments (with numbers, if possible: increases in sales or share of market, cost-cutting, profitability, etc.).
- Match the language of the job posting, especially when referring to the position you're applying for.
- Include a LinkedIn profile.
- Put your education at the end and omit graduation dates.

- Keep it to one or two pages.
- Ditch outdated formatting and font styles. Have a single font, preferably sans serif in 10 or 12 point, and keep it consistent throughout the résumé. You don't need your entire address, just email and phone, but make sure your email isn't in an older domain like AOL or Hotmail. Get a Gmail account instead.

IN THE MARKETPLACE

Although an individual may be relatively ineffective when calling out against ageism in the broader culture ("OK, Boomer," etc.), the same is not true when it comes to fighting against ageism in the marketplace. Here the individual SuperAger may have, if anything, outsized influence.

In the highly politicized environment of today, many advertisers are hypersensitive to consumer complaints, and there are regulatory agencies on the lookout for abuses in marketing and advertising. Groups that have been historically underrepresented in advertising (people of color, LGBTQ, mixed-race couples, to name a few) have been very successful in getting the advertising community to cast more of their members in ads and commercials—a development that can only be applauded.

Consider what has been accomplished. The underrepresentation of these groups had nothing to do with misleading product claims or other fraudulent practices—the traditional grounds for complaints against advertising that have numerous forms of relief through regulatory agencies or tort law. The protests against underrepresentation had to do with racial and social justice, with a moral obligation on the part of advertisers to accurately reflect the makeup of society. Casting more members of underrepresented groups in ads and commercials was seen as an important step toward diversity and inclusion. The advertising community has been quick to respond to this critique.

There is no reason why the pressure cannot be exerted to combat ageism. Instead of just bemoaning it, SuperAgers can push back forcefully. It is important to realize that a relatively small number of protests can have an outsized effect precisely because corporations and their ad agencies are in an extremely sensitive (and, frankly, defensive) mode at the moment.

SuperAgers who see an ad or commercial that displays ageism should consider the following menu of responses:

File a formal complaint with regulators. In the United States, the Federal Communications Commission regulates mass media, and the Federal Trade Commission also has a role in policing misleading advertising. In Canada, there is a variety of federal and provincial agencies, depending on the media used and the products being advertised (e.g., health products can fall under the Health Canada ministry). Also, an industry association, the Ad Standards Council, will receive complaints. In the United Kingdom, there exists a wide range of regulations and controls, plus a mix of government supervisory bodies and industry self-regulatory groups. Check our Resources section at SuperAging.info for a list of key websites.

File a complaint with the media where you saw the ad or commercial. Let them know that by running this ad or commercial, they are supporting ageism. Send a copy of your letter to the appropriate regulatory body and post it to the internet in any social media channel you're involved with, encouraging all your friends to circulate it as well. All media have internal review processes under which they can accept or reject a given ad or commercial; the goal here is to embarrass them into declining to run the offending ad or commercial in the future. Your copy to the regulatory body will increase the anxiety for the media in question, as the last thing they want is an official inquiry into why they are promoting ageism.

Stop purchasing the product. Write a letter to the chief marketing officer of the company that ran the offending ad or commercial, explaining your decision. Add that you are mobilizing all your friends to stop buying the product. Be sure to send a copy of the letter to the president of the company and, if it's a public company, to the chairperson of the board. (Note: The average tenure of a CMO is now only 40 months, the lowest level it has reached in over a decade. The last thing the CMO needs is to attract the attention of higher-ups on the grounds of having promoted ageism.) Remember, too, that SuperAgers are the largest and wealthiest cohort of consumers in the marketplace, and don't hesitate to place that factoid very prominently in your letter.

It may seem strange to you that we're making this kind of recommendation since both of us have spent our professional careers in the marketing communications industry. But that's precisely the point. We know how the industry works; we know what they're afraid of.

We also admire the many advertisers who do get it and don't promote ageism. Many skin-care and cosmetics brands, for example, have featured SuperAger celebrity spokespeople. Susan Sarandon represented Revlon in 2005, when she was 58. In 2014, L'Oréal signed Helen Mirren, then 69. Joan Collins was 86 (not a typo!) when she became the "face" of Charlotte Tilbury in 2019. So it can be done. Which is our whole point: It is perfectly fair to push, and push hard, against those who aren't doing it. In terms of their purchasing power, SuperAgers already control the marketplace; if they raise their voices against ageism in that marketplace—and especially if they threaten to withhold that purchasing power—they will definitely be heard.

AVOIDING FRAUDS AND SCAMS

There are three simple strategies here:

1. Know what techniques are out there.
2. Know where to report a fraud, scam, or security breach if you think it's happened to you.
3. Build a defensive wall in the digital space.

The first item is important simply because the scammers' range of weapons is constantly being updated and expanded. They're also very quick to develop cons that play into other current issues—COVID was a classic example. There are over 40,000 domain names with the word "covid" or "coronavirus," so links to these sources or emails coming from them have the look of legitimacy. Yet many, if not most, are from scammers. Techniques include fake products like masks, fake test kits, or fake online tests (just click on the link to register for the test—but now the scammer has access to your computer). There's even outright blackmail: with so many people now using videoconferencing software like Zoom or Google Meet, scammers have been sending out mass emails advising the targets that their web camera has been hacked and that intimate, compromising video has been captured and will be circulated to all friends and colleagues until a ransom is paid . . . in Bitcoin.

We recommend periodically checking with organizations like AARP or CARP, who regularly report on the latest frauds and scams, and who in turn can link you to appropriate local resources, including law enforcement agencies who keep up to date and often issue advisories.

For the second item—where to report—the simplest answer is to alert your local police, who will know how to handle your complaint or to which other enforcement agency to route it. Since many frauds and scams may involve bank accounts or credit cards, any known (or even suspicious) activity should be reported immediately to the banks or credit card companies. Every credit agency and bank also maintains their own security operation with sophisticated algorithms to monitor transactions and flag unusual or potentially fraudulent activity. The good news here is that there is a strong support system in place; the key is to react promptly.

For the final item of building your virtual defenses, there is a lot of direct action that should be taken:

- Install a strong antivirus, anti-malware program on your computer and smartphone. Set up automatic daily scans of your computer's hard drive.
- *Never* click on a link on an inbound email or text message unless you are 100% certain of who the sender is and what the link is about. Even then, it doesn't hurt to verify that it was truly sent by that sender.
- Be particularly vigilant about emails whose subject lines state that you have won a prize or can receive an instant reward for completing a survey, or that a delivery to you has been delayed and needs reconfirmation. When you receive such emails, don't just ignore them; set up a filter to automatically delete them in the future.
- Don't answer any inbound phone call that shows just a phone number and no caller ID. There may be a very few exceptions, such as if you know the caller, but the general rule of thumb should be: if you can't see who's calling, don't take the call. Even better, program your smartphone to block that number in the future.

- Consider an identity theft protection program.
  There are many services that can patrol the internet,
  including the dark web, to see if your Social Security
  number, bank accounts, or credit cards have been
  compromised.

Fighting frauds and scams is, unfortunately, grunt work—an ongoing grind rather than a single overarching strategy. It means paying attention to a lot of nasty little things. But increasingly, there are many tech solutions that can help. Frauds and scams can be avoided, but the necessary homework can't.

AVOIDING OBSOLETE ADVISERS

With the best intentions in the world, doctors, financial planners, and other advisers may not offer the best counsel because they're still trapped in the DefaultAging mode of thinking. This can lead to what we might call soft forms of ageism: spending less time with you than they should, dismissing your concerns, or not really understanding how you view the future (especially if your viewpoint is different from theirs). The result is not so much their offering blatant, disastrously wrong advice—doing X instead of Y—but rather, a slow and creeping failure to take maximum advantage of new approaches and opportunities.

We recommend an audit, through the SuperAging lens, of the adviser's knowledge and approach. This can be as simple as asking yourself a series of questions without ever having a dialogue with the adviser. Or it can be a frank one-on-one session where you really probe what the adviser knows and thinks.

CHECKLIST FOR EVALUATING YOUR DOCTOR

Here we're only talking about the GP or family physician, your first line of medical assessment and the gatekeeper to the entire system. It would be presumptuous, to the point of irresponsible, to offer generalized advice about dealing with specialists who may be treating serious conditions. But for the family physician, it is not unreasonable to undertake an audit of the doctor's knowledge and approach. Key questions to consider:

- **What is the doctor's overall attitude?** Is the doctor arrogant or condescending? There may have been a time when you needed to accept this; that time has passed.
- **Are they a good listener?** If not, this is another sign of ageism: your views don't matter, the doctor is the pro, let's just hurry things along.
- **Is each visit a separate and distinct event or part of a continuum?** In DefaultAging, the transaction model prevailed. You got sick, you went to the doctor, you got better, you didn't see the doctor again until the next time you were sick. Is that how your doctor treats each visit? Is the doctor aware of your overall treatment history, or any patterns? Is your chart readily available on the doctor's computer screen? Do they ever act as if not 100% sure who you are?
- **How do they respond to your concerns?** Is your doctor interested in or dismissive of information or ideas you yourself may be advancing? Are you afraid to bring up something you saw on the internet? Are you nervous about mentioning things like supplements or alternative therapies?
- **Are they aware of emerging new technologies for**

diagnostics and better patient service? Telehealth, wireless trackers, electronic health records, technology to make it easier for you to age at home . . . Does it look/sound/feel like your doctor is up to date on the current state of play and where it's going?

- **Do they have any idea about your future potential and your actual plans?** This is another aspect of a one-shot transaction versus a continuum of care. Does your doctor think you are a SuperAger? Do they even know what that is? Have they ever shown any interest in what you might be up to in 5 or 10 years—and what the healthcare implications are for that goal? Or is it always just the immediate issue of today's visit?

- **If you were a customer instead of a patient, how would your doctor stack up?** Do the appointments start on time? Is the facility clean and bright, the supporting staff friendly? Taking the whole package together as one, is it an enterprise that understands you and your needs, and that is motivated to deliver outstanding service? Thinking like a consumer, would you rather take your business elsewhere?

CHECKLIST FOR EVALUATING YOUR FINANCIAL ADVISER

The situation with a financial adviser is a bit different than with a doctor. In the first place, you can get, if you want it, a daily (or even hourly) readout of how you're doing, and you may well decide to put up with a certain degree of less-than-stellar service as long as the numbers remain good. So it's not for us to casually advise any individual SuperAger to fire their financial adviser!

Second, consumerism has always been a factor, to some degree, in the financial services industry. There are plenty of advisers, both stand-alone planners and planners attached to banks, credit unions, and other financial institutions. There is also a long history of marketing to consumers based not only on (real or perceived) knowledge of the economy and investments but also on the ability to understand the individual investor's needs and tailor a plan for them. Of course, there is a wide range of actual performance outcomes, but at least the industry presents itself as concerned, involved, and service oriented, whereas the medical profession is comparatively less so.

The chances are good, therefore, that a SuperAger's financial adviser has already proved themself, to some degree, over the years and in varying market conditions.

But it still makes sense to conduct an audit (even if only a dialogue with yourself) similar to what we recommended above for doctors. What you're after here is not so much stock-picking ability, but breadth of knowledge about the many new financial challenges and opportunities generated by the SuperAging revolution. Does the adviser have a wide-enough horizon?

You could form those judgments yourself, based on your experience with that financial adviser. You could also ask the adviser some pointed questions like these:

- Are you aware of my future career plans?
  - Would it surprise you to learn that I'm planning to retire at 65 / keep working past 65 / shift to an entirely new career or activity?
  - How do you think that would influence the financial program we've developed together?
- Are you aware of my current housing situation and its suitability/unsuitability for aging in place?
  - Would it surprise you to learn that I want to age

in place and not go into a retirement residence or community (let alone a long-term care facility)?

- Do you think I can stay in my current home?
- Do you have an idea of changes or upgrades I should make, and what they would cost?
- Are you able to map out those costs over an extended period of time (perhaps decades)?
- Do you think that knowledge on this topic should be considered as part of your responsibilities?
- Are you aware of new interests or activities I'm engaged in?
  - How much do you really know about me, other than how my portfolio is doing?
- Do you believe I should evaluate my financial program based on the same criteria as we've used in the past?
  - What about issues like outliving my money and the need for income?
  - What about cash flow and not just ROI?
  - Does longevity mean I can actually have a slightly higher tolerance for risk?
- Are you aware of SuperAging?
  - Even if you don't know about the exact phrase, how aware are you of longevity and its implications for financial planning?
  - Some of the most exciting developments in extending the human life span will involve higher costs. How can we make sure that I'll be in a position to afford the new drugs or high-tech solutions?
- Have you taken any steps to improve or upgrade your knowledge and skills as they specifically relate to the topic of aging?

- Have you taken any training programs and obtained a seniors designation or certification of any kind?
- Do you think you need more expertise on your team to really help me?
  - Do you see yourself, in the future, as the quarterback of a team that can bring more experience and expertise to the issue? Can you bring in a real estate specialist if required? An occupational therapist who can audit my home for its aging-in-place potential and map out a plan for renovation? A high-tech expert? A lifestyle reinvention coach? Or is it up to me to find these people?

The answers to these questions will give you a lot of insight into how well your planner is equipped—in terms of both abilities and attitudes—to meet your future needs as a SuperAger. In addition, there is the issue of customer service, and you should evaluate this against the same ageism yardsticks that were applied to your family doctor. Good warning signs that it's time to say goodbye:

- Your planner is a poor listener.
- Your planner is casual about service (hard to get hold of, vague about explaining fees).
- Your planner is dismissive or patronizing about your concerns and treats them as something you shouldn't trouble yourself with.

9

YOU'RE A SUPERAGER NOW!

Congratulations! With these seven pillars, you now have the program you need to become part of the SuperAging revolution. Now you'll be able to get older without getting old!

Is there a lot to do? Well, there's certainly a lot to pay attention to. But hopefully we've been able to boil it down into a logical and manageable list. You may choose simply to keep an eye on that list and measure your own actions and responses informally. Or you may prefer to go into much more detail and set up a formal action plan and system of to-do lists. Your response to the SuperAging opportunity, especially at the beginning, can be flexible and tailored to your specific needs and preferences.

The most important point is: You have a new perspective. (To check that new perspective, here's your reminder to redo the quizzes you took in the chapter on Attitude.)

It *is* possible to live much longer. And it *is* possible to experience those extra years as a time of growth, development, and accomplishment as opposed to decline and retreat. What's more, that growth and development is made even more exciting precisely because of the lifetime of learning and experience you've already gained. That's why we make no apology for the "age" part of SuperAging. It's not something to hide or work around; it's an essential component to making the future so rich. Your accumulated knowledge and wisdom (including the mistakes you've learned from) are priceless building blocks for a future that has plenty of capacity to be even more fulfilling.

It's exciting to be a SuperAger!

You're part of a worldwide community now, a community that is carrying out the most profound and far-reaching social development in history: the redefinition of aging itself.

We encourage you to keep that idea of community firmly in your mind as you tap into the opportunities we provide. This book is only the first step. As we've mentioned throughout, our companion website, SuperAging.info, is an essential component as well. SuperAging is a topic around which something new is happening all the time—new research and discoveries, new products and services, new ways to meet like-minded people—and the internet is obviously the best way to stay updated. SuperAging.info will offer more detailed resources for the topics we've covered here, as well as news, podcasts, videos (also see our YouTube channel!), interviews with experts, and an entire interactive community where you, as a SuperAger, can share information and ideas with other SuperAgers.

Thank you for embracing SuperAging. It's going to be an exciting future for all of us!

ACKNOWLEDGMENTS

David and Larry are grateful for the tremendous support we've received from our publishers, Flashpoint Books, and the editorial and design team at Girl Friday Productions: Kristin Mehus-Roe, Sara Addicott, Adria Batt, and Jaye Whitney Debber. Special kudos to our developmental editor, Marisa Solis, who brought a unique mix of tough-minded insistence on clarity and quality and sympathetic appreciation of our "voice" and what we were trying to do. We were truly fortunate to be in the hands of such an enthusiastic and skilled team!

David wants to acknowledge the tremendous contribution of my wife, Cynthia, who has been both an inspiration and a no-nonsense advocate for "You can still make this better." As with my previous books, I have relied on her knowledge and wisdom. I also appreciate the support of my colleagues at ZoomerMedia, particularly our CEO, Moses Znaimer, who is always a source of new ideas and an encourager of new possibilities, and Libby Znaimer, who conducted a one-hour interview with me, on national TV, prior to the book being published. Your support and endorsement are deeply appreciated.

Larry wants to acknowledge the tremendous support and contribution of my wife, Mary. Mary, one of the smartest communications professionals I know, has a unique ability to articulate the perspective of the reader. Her incisive criticisms and insights were invaluable in developing our book.

REFERENCES

1. THE 7A'S OF SUPERAGING

Blumberg, Yoni. "Millennials Spend Less Than Previous
   Generations Because They Literally Have Less Money,
   Fed Says." CNBC, December 4, 2018. https://www.cnbc
   .com/2018/12/04/millennials-spend-less-because-theyre
   -poorer-federal-reserve-says.html.

Clark, Amie. "Life on a College or University Campus—an
   Alternative Retirement Destination." Senior List, April 1,
   2022. https://www.theseniorlist.com/retirement/best
   /university/.

Pawlowski, A. "Optimists Live Longer, Study Finds. Here's
   How to Boost Positive Thinking." *Today*, August 26, 2019.
   https://www.today.com/health/how-live-longer-study
   -links-optimism-longevity-t161337.

2. ATTITUDE

Alimujiang, Aliya, Ashley Wiensch, Jonathan Boss, et al.
   "Association Between Life Purpose and Mortality Among
   US Adults Older Than 50 Years." JAMA Network (May 24,
   2019). https://jamanetwork.com/journals/jamanetworkopen
   /fullarticle/2734064.

BU School of Medicine. "New Evidence That Optimists Live
   Longer." August 26, 2019. https://www.bumc.bu.edu
   /busm/2019/08/26/new-evidence-that-optimists-live-longer/.

Christensen, Kaare, Anne Maria Herskind, and James W.
    Vaupel. "Why Danes Are Smug: Comparative Study of Life
    Satisfaction in the European Union." *BMJ* 333, no. 7582
    (2006): 1289–91. https://www.ncbi.nlm.nih.gov/pmc/articles
    /PMC1761170/.

Cravit, David. "J. P. Morgan Tells Its Advisors to Assume
    Retirees Will Live to 100." Everything Zoomer, April 18,
    2022. https://www.everythingzoomer.com/health/longevity
    -wellness/2022/04/18/j-p-morgan-tells-its-advisors-to
    -assume-retirees-will-live-to-100.

Fielding, Sarah. "Why 1 in 5 Adults Over Age 50 Say Their Sex
    Life Is Way More Exciting Now." *mbgRelationships*, June 23,
    2019. https://www.mindbodygreen.com/articles/how-often
    -people-have-sex-after-50-60-70-and-older-and-how-to
    -increase-frequency/.

Fogelman, Nia, and Turhan Canli. "'Purpose in Life' as a
    Psychosocial Resource in Healthy Aging: An Examination
    of Cortisol Baseline Levels and Response to the Trier Social
    Stress Test." *npj Aging*, September 28, 2015. https://www
    .nature.com/articles/npjamd20156.

Gander, Kashmira. "Religious People Live Four Years Longer
    on Average: Study." *Newsweek*, June 14, 2018. https://www
    .newsweek.com/religious-people-live-four-years-longer
    -average-study-shows-976050.

Hall, Nicholas. "Is Feeling Better as Easy as ABC?" *Positive
    Psychology News*, June 6, 2007. https://positivepsychologynews
    .com/news/nicholas-hall/20070606273.

Hayes, Kim. "How Is Your Emodiversity?" *AARP*, June 27, 2017.
    https://www.aarp.org/health/conditions-treatments/info
    -2017/positive-emotions-may-reduce-inflammation-fd.html.

Hennefield, Laura, Laura M. Talpey, and Lori Markson. "When
    Positive Outcomes and Reality Collide: Children Prefer
    Optimists as Social Partners." *Cognitive Development* 59

(2021). https://www.ncbi.nlm.nih.gov/pmc/articles
/PMC8478345/.

Klein, Jessica. "Are Baby Boomers Having the Best Time in
Bed?" *BBC News*, April 21, 2022. https://www.bbc.com
/worklife/article/20220420-are-baby-boomers-having-the
-best-time-in-bed.

Mathur, Maya B., Elissa Epel, Shelley Kind, Manisha Desai,
Christine G. Parks, Dale P. Sandler, and Nayer Khazeni.
"Perceived Stress and Telomere Length: A Systematic
Review, Meta-analysis, and Methodologic Considerations
for Advancing the Field." *Brain, Behavior, and Immunity* 54
(May 2016): 158–69. https://www.sciencedirect.com/science
/article/pii/S088915911630023X?via%3Dihub.

Plomin, Richard, Michael F. Scheier, C. S. Bergeman, N. L.
Pedersen, J. R. Nesselroade, and G. E. McClearn. "Optimism,
Pessimism, and Mental Health: A Twin/Adoption Analysis."
Personality and Individual Differences 13, no. 8 (August
1992): 921–30. https://www.sciencedirect.com/science
/article/abs/pii/019188699290009E.

Robson, David. "Can You Think Yourself Young?" *Guardian*,
January 2, 2022. https://www.theguardian.com/science/2022
/jan/02/can-you-think-yourself-young-ageing-psychology.

Rosenthal, Jack. "Language: What Will You Call Me When I'm
64?" *New York Times*, July 27, 2007. https://www.nytimes
.com/2007/07/22/opinion/22iht-edrosenthal.1.6767016.html.

Skipper, Clay. "Why Your Brain Is Wired for Pessimism—and
What You Can Do to Fix It." *GQ*, September 23, 2018.
https://www.gq.com/story/how-to-be-more-optimistic.

Tessler Lindau, Stacy, et al. "A Study of Sexuality and Health
Among Older Adults in the United States." *New England
Journal of Medicine*, August 23, 2007. https://www.nejm.org
/doi/full/10.1056/nejmoa067423.

"Thinking Positively About Aging Extends Life More Than

Exercise and Not Smoking." *YaleNews*, July 29, 2002. https://news.yale.edu/2002/07/29/thinking-positively-about-aging-extends-life-more-exercise-and-not-smoking.

University of Kansas. "People by Nature Are Universally Optimistic, Study Shows." *ScienceDaily*, May 25, 2009. https://www.sciencedaily.com/releases/2009/05/090524122539.htm.

4. ACTIVITY

Baker, Joseph, et al. "Sport Participation and Positive Development in Older Persons." *European Review of Aging and Physical Activity* 7 (2010). https://eurapa.biomedcentral.com/articles/10.1007/s11556-009-0054-9.

Browse by Collection. DIYbiosphere, 2022. https://sphere.diybio.org/.

Bryant, Erin. "Lack of Sleep in Middle Age May Increase Dementia Risk." National Institutes of Health, April 27, 2021. https://www.nih.gov/news-events/nih-research-matters/lack-sleep-middle-age-may-increase-dementia-risk.

Elhuyar Foundation. "Study on 90-Year-Olds Reveals the Benefits of Strength Training." *ScienceDaily*, September 27, 2013. https://www.sciencedaily.com/releases/2013/09/130927092350.htm#.

"From Grinders to Biohackers: Where Medical Technology Meets Body Modification." *Medical Technology*, January 2022. https://medical-technology.nridigital.com/medical_technology_jan20/from_grinders_to_biohackers_where_medical_technology_meets_body_modification.

Healthline Editorial Team. "Why It's Never Too Late to Start Exercising." *Healthline*, September 4, 2019. https://www.healthline.com/health-news/why-its-never-too-late-to-start-exercising.

Herskind, Anne Maria, Matt Mcgue, Niels Vilstrup Holm, and Thorkild I. A. Sørensen. "The Heritability of Human Longevity: A Population-Based Study of 2,872 Danish Twin Pairs Born 1870–1900." *Human Genetics* 97, no. 3 (April 1996): 319–23. https://www.researchgate.net /publication/14416947_The_heritability_of_human _longevity_A_population-based_study_of_2872_Danish _twin_pairs_born_1870-1900.

Huang, Jiaqi, et al. "Association Between Plant and Animal Protein Intake and Overall and Cause-Specific Mortality." *JAMA Internal Medicine* 180, no. 9 (2020): 1173–84. https:// pubmed.ncbi.nlm.nih.gov/32658243/.

Klatsky, Arthur L. "Moderate Drinking and Reduced Risk of Heart Disease." *Alcohol Research & Health* 23, no. 1 (1999): 15–24. https://www.ncbi.nlm.nih.gov/pmc/articles /PMC6761693/.

LaCroix, Andrea Z., et al. "Does Walking Decrease the Risk of Cardiovascular Disease Hospitalizations and Death in Older Adults?" *Journal of the American Geriatrics Society* 44, no. 2 (February 1996): 113–20. https://agsjournals.onlinelibrary .wiley.com/doi/abs/10.1111/j.1532-5415.1996.tb02425.x.

Lanza, Ian R., et al. "Chronic Caloric Restriction Preserves Mitochondrial Function in Senescence Without Increasing Mitochondrial Biogenesis." *Cell Metabolism* 16, no. 6 (2012): 777–78. https://www.ncbi.nlm.nih.gov/pmc/articles /PMC3544078/.

Lineaweaver, Nicky. "Patients Are Transforming from Passive Recipients of Healthcare Services to Active Participants in Their Own Health." *Yahoo! News*, July 11, 2019. https:// news.yahoo.com/patients-transforming-passive-recipients -healthcare-050000224.html.

Maki, Jessica. "Berries Delay Memory Decline in Adults." *SciTechDaily*, April 27, 2012. https://scitechdaily.com /berries-delay-memory-decline-in-adults/.

Mazzotti, Diego Robles, et al. "Human Longevity Is Associated with Regular Sleep Patterns, Maintenance of Slow Wave Sleep, and Favorable Lipid Profile." *Frontiers in Aging Neuroscience* 6, no. 134 (2014). https://www.ncbi.nlm.nih .gov/pmc/articles/PMC4067693/.

McKeehan, Nick. "Loneliness and the Risk of Dementia." *Cognitive Vitality* (blog), April 16, 2019. https://www .alzdiscovery.org/cognitive-vitality/blog/loneliness-and -the-risk-of-dementia.

Murez, Cara. "This Balance Test May Predict Longevity." *HealthDay*, June 22, 2022. https://www.medicinenet.com /script/main/art.asp?articlekey=278013.

"Nutrigenomics: The Basics." Nutrition Society, November 19, 2018. https://www.nutritionsociety.org/blog /nutrigenomics-basics.

Physicians Committee for Responsible Medicine. "Consuming More Protein from Plants Associated with Longer Life." *Health and Nutrition News*, July 23, 2020. https://www.pcrm.org/news/health-nutrition /consuming-more-protein-plants-associated-longer-life.

Reynolds, Gretchen. "Brisk Walking Is Good for the Aging Brain." *New York Times*, March 31, 2021. https://www .nytimes.com/2021/03/31/well/move/seniors-memory -walking.html.

———. "Walking Just 10 Minutes a Day May Lead to a Longer Life." *New York Times*, January 26, 2022. https://www .nytimes.com/2022/01/26/well/10-minutes-walking-exercise .html#.

Robertson, Sally. "Walking for Just 20 Minutes a Day May Reduce Death Risk." *News Medical Life Sciences*, January 15, 2015. https://www.news-medical.net/news/20150115 /Walking-for-just-20-minutes-a-day-may-reduce-death-risk .aspx.

Stenner, Brad J., Jonathan D. Buckley, and Amber D. Mosewich. "Reasons Why Older Adults Play Sport: A Systematic Review." *Journal of Sport and Health Science* 9, no. 6 (2020): 530–41. https://pubmed.ncbi.nlm.nih.gov/33308804/.

"Study Finds Association Between Sleep Problems and Dementia." National Heart, Lung, and Blood Institute, July 2, 2021. https://www.nhlbi.nih.gov/news/2021/study-finds-association-between-sleep-problems-and-dementia#.

Van Gelder, B. M., et al. "Coffee Consumption Is Inversely Associated with Cognitive Decline in Elderly European Men: The FINE Study." *European Journal of Clinical Nutrition* 61, no. 2 (2007): 226–32. https://pubmed.ncbi.nlm.nih.gov/16929246/.

Zylberberg, Shawn. "Aiming to Live Past 90? Moderate Wine Consumption Could Help." *Wine Spectator*, March 4, 2020. https://www.winespectator.com/articles/aiming-to-live-past-90-moderate-wine-consumption-could-help#.

7. ATTACHMENT

University of Chicago. "Loneliness Triggers Cellular Changes That Can Cause Illness, Study Shows." *ScienceDaily*, November 23, 2015. https://www.sciencedaily.com/releases/2015/11/151123201925.htm.

8. AVOIDANCE

Levy, Becca R., et al. "Ageism Amplifies Cost and Prevalence of Health Conditions." *Gerontologist* 60, no. 1 (February 2020): 174–81. https://academic.oup.com/gerontologist/article/60/1/174/5166947.

Martin, Ashley, and Michael S. North. "Equality for (Almost)
    All: Egalitarian Advocacy Predicts Lower Endorsement of
    Sexism and Racism, but Not Ageism." *Journal of Personality
    and Social Psychology* 123, no. 2 (January 2021). https://
    www.researchgate.net/publication/348609257_Equality
    _for_almost_all_Egalitarian_advocacy_predicts_lower
    _endorsement_of_sexism_and_racism_but_not_ageism.

ABOUT THE AUTHORS

David Cravit has an established profile and track record in reporting on aging and related issues. He is the author of two previous books: *The New Old*, which discusses how the Baby Boomers reinvented aging, and *Beyond Age Rage*, which examines the so-called war of the generations. He is a vice president at ZoomerMedia, the only media company in Canada specializing in the "older" market, and also chief membership officer and chief marketing officer of CARP (Canada's equivalent to AARP). He appears frequently on radio and television as a respected commentator on the new trends and developments driving the emergence of SuperAging.

Larry Wolf's expertise is in identifying important trends and creating opportunities to capitalize on them. He has advised a number of *Fortune* 500 companies and governments on their branding and communications strategies. Larry founded and developed the Wolf Group from a two-person consultancy into a sizable international advertising agency with offices in seven cities in the United States and Canada. His company helped successfully create and launch many new brands. Most recently, Larry identified a number of trends precipitated by increasing longevity and made use of an unrealized opportunity to unify and brand the key elements that contribute to successful aging.